NATIONAL FORUM ON HEALTH / FORUM NATIONAL SUR LA SANTÉ

Canada Health Action: Building on the Legacy

Volume II

Synthesis Reports and Issues Papers

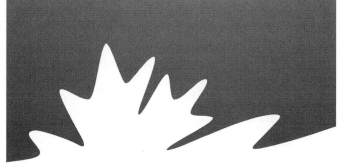

Canada

The complete report of the National Forum on Health comprises:

Volume I -   Canada Health Action: Building on the Legacy
              The Final Report of the National Forum on Health

Volume II -   Canada Health Action: Building on the Legacy
              Synthesis Reports and Issues Papers
              Values Working Group Synthesis Report
              Determinants of Health Working Group Synthesis Report
              Striking a Balance Working Group Synthesis Report
              Creating a Culture of Evidence-Based Decision Making

              The Need for an Aboriginal Health Institute in Canada
              Directions for a Pharmaceutical Policy in Canada
              An Overview of Women's Health

As well, the Forum will publish the papers commissioned in the course of its work.
The publication of these papers (1997) will provide Canadians with a considerable amount of
research in the field of health and health care in Canada.

The Report of the National Forum on Health is also available on Internet and in alternative format.

Published by:
National Forum on Health
P.O. Box 2798
4th Floor, 200 Kent Street
Ottawa, Ontario
K1P 6H4

Fax: (613) 954-0947
e-mail: forum@hpb.hwc.ca
www: http://wwwnfh.hwc.ca

Cat. No. H21-126/5-2-1997E
ISBN   0-662-25306-X

Aussi disponible en français.

Contents

Introduction

Values Working Group Synthesis Report

Striking a Balance Working Group Synthesis Report

Determinants of Health Working Group Synthesis Report

Creating a Culture of Evidence-Based Decision Making

The Need for an Aboriginal Health Institute in Canada

Directions for a Pharmaceutical Policy in Canada

An Overview of Women's Health

Appendix: National Forum on Health Publications

Introduction

The National Forum on Health is pleased to present *Canada Health Action: Building on the Legacy, Synthesis Reports and Issues Papers,* (Volume II of the Final Report). This document presents the detailed analysis and rationale, as well as recommendations, that led to the Forum's priorities, outlined in Volume I.

In October 1994, the Prime Minister of Canada, The Right Honourable Jean Chrétien, launched the National Forum on Health to involve and inform Canadians and to advise the federal government on innovative ways to improve our health system and the health of Canada's people. The Forum was set up as an advisory body with the Prime Minister as Chair, the federal Minister of Health as Vice Chair, and 24 volunteer members who contributed a wide range of knowledge founded on involvement in the health system as professionals, consumers and volunteers.

To fulfil our mandate, the Forum focused on long-term and systemic issues. We saw our task as formulating advice appropriate to the development of national policies, and we divided our work into four key areas — Values, Striking a Balance, Determinants of Health, and Evidence-Based Decision Making. This document contains the individual synthesis papers developed by each of the Forum working groups on these key areas, as well as issue specific papers on an Aboriginal Health Institute, pharmaceuticals and women's health.

Values

The Values working group sought to understand the values and principles that Canadians hold about health and health care, so that the system continues to reflect and respond to these values. To explore Canadian core values that are connected to the health care system and to understand the implications for decision making, the group conducted some original public opinion research, using scenarios or short stories which addressed many of the issues being investigated by the other working groups of the Forum. The scenarios were tested in focus groups. Quantitative research supplemented the focus groups making the findings more generalizable. The group also contributed to a review of public opinion research on health and social policy. Finally, a review of Canadian and international experience with ethics bodies was commissioned to identify the contribution that such groups can make to continuing the discussion of values in decision making. The *Values Working Group Synthesis Report* presents the results of this work, and the analysis and conclusions of the working group.

Striking a Balance

This group considered how to allocate society's limited resources to best protect, restore and promote the health of Canadians. Attention was given to the balance of resources within the health sector, and between the health sector and other sectors of the economy. The group commissioned a series of papers to assist in their deliberations. They conducted a thorough review of international trends in health expenditures, use of resources, and outcomes. They paid considerable attention to public and private financing issues, health system organization and federal-provincial transfers. The group produced a separate discussion paper on public and private financing, and a position paper on the Canada Health and Social Transfer. The *Striking a Balance Working Group Synthesis Report* contains the analysis, conclusions and recommendations which the group has drawn from this commissioned work, their deliberations, and the Forum's discussion process.

Determinants of Health

The Determinants of Health working group sought to answer the question, In these times of economic and social hardship, what actions must be taken to allow Canadians to continue to enjoy a long life and, if possible, to increase their health status? The group consulted specialists to assist in identifying appropriate actions on the non-medical determinants of health. Specialists were asked to prepare papers on issues of concern to the health of the population related to the macro-economic environment, the contexts in which people live (i.e. families, schools, work and communities), as well as on issues of concern to people's health at different life stages. Each paper presents a review of the literature, examples of success stories or failures, and relevant policy implications. The working group also drew from the consultations with the public and with stakeholders in arriving at the analysis, conclusions and recommendations which are presented in the *Determinants of Health Working Group Synthesis Report*.

Evidence-Based Decision Making

The working group on Evidence-Based Decision Making considered how individuals, practitioners and policy makers can have access to, and utilize the best available evidence in making decisions. The group held two workshops with leading authorities to discuss how health information can be used to support and encourage a culture of evidence-based decision making, and to consider what information Canadians need to be better health care consumers and how to get that information to them. The group commissioned papers to: examine the meaning and concepts of evidence and evidence-based decision making; identify cases of successful implementation of evidence-based decision making as well as cases that illustrate opportunities for improvement; identify the health information infrastructure needed to support evidence-based decision making; examine tools which support more effective health care decision making; and identify strategies for assisting and increasing the role of Canadians in decision making in health and health care. The group's synthesis report, *Creating a Culture of Evidence-Based Decision Making*, contains the analysis, conclusions and recommendations resulting from the group's consideration of these papers, and the Forum's extensive consultations and deliberations.

An Aboriginal Health Institute

Aboriginal health issues were considered by each working group, as part of their respective mandates. In addition, a small group of Forum members considered the contribution that the Forum could make to improving the health of Aboriginal peoples. The paper titled *The Need for an Aboriginal Health Institute* is the result of Forum deliberations.

Pharmaceutical Policy

Two working groups—Striking a Balance and Evidence-Based Decision Making—jointly considered issues pertaining to pharmaceuticals. The paper, *Directions for a Pharmaceutical Policy in Canada,* results from their deliberations.

Women's Health

The papers commissioned for the Determinants of Health working group, together with the findings from the Forum's consultations and papers from the Canada - US Forum on Women's Health, were reviewed to highlight key aspects and issues about women's health. The results of this review are summarized in the paper, *An Overview of Women's Health*.

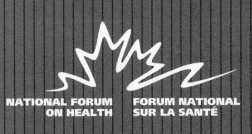

NATIONAL FORUM
ON HEALTH

FORUM NATIONAL
SUR LA SANTÉ

Values
Working
Group
Synthesis
Report

Values Working Group

Nuala Kenny, M.D. (Chair)
Randy Dickinson
Madeleine Dion Stout, M.A.
Richard Lessard, M.D.
Gerry Lougheed Jr.
Shanthi Radcliffe, M.A.
Duncan Sinclair, Ph.D.

John Dossetor (Policy Analyst)

Contents

Introduction 3

Key Findings 5

    Canadians value their health system 5

Concern for the Future 9

Canadian Pride and National Identity 10

The Twin Pillars of Access and Quality 12

Support for Change that Increases Efficiency and Effectiveness 14

Investing in Disease Prevention and Health Promotion 15

The Expanding Spectrum of Health Care Services 17

Care Closer to the Home 18

Ethical Reflection in Canada 20

Conclusions 22

References 25

Appendix A 26

Appendix B 36

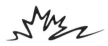

Introduction

There has been much public discussion about the need to reform the health system but correspondingly little discussion of the importance and significance of underlying societal values in the health reform agenda. We know little about the impact of large scale health reform on our individual experiences and our publicly held values.

In the face of reform of the health system in Canada, a number of difficult questions have arisen. For example, do we as a population want increased privatization of our health system, greater freedom of choice, increased commitment to care in the home and greater investment in the wider determinants of health? Do we think that certain policies should take precedence over others? Is one policy alternative more in keeping with our values than another? These are some of the questions currently being asked in our society and which should be answered not solely on the basis of cost consideration, but with due regard to the opinions, beliefs and values held by Canadians. With this in mind, the National Forum on Health formed the working group on Values to investigate and report on how and what Canadians think about these and other issues relating to health and the Canadian health care system.

The Values Working Group intends to contribute to a national dialogue by identifying those values and principles which Canadians hold regarding health and the health care system.

The National Forum on Health is in itself an expression of the importance of the values of dialogue, participation and respectful listening. It is not an expert panel, nor is it a process in which the majority wins.

Understanding the nature of Canadian opinion and underlying values will assist in refining policy recommendations to reflect better views and concerns that Canadians have regarding health and health care. For a new vision to be acceptable by Canadians, it must resonate with the values accepted as relevant, valid and important in their lives. Not all Canadians share the same values nor are all these values amenable to change. Policy recommendations of the National Forum on Health will not be accepted by all Canadians on all issues. However, it is essential that Canadians know that their values have been heard and understood by the Forum.

For a new vision to be acceptable by Canadians, it must resonate with the values accepted as relevant, valid and important in their lives.

The Values Working Group is of the opinion that understanding the "landscape" is a critical step before trying to recommend a route for the future. The "landscape" is not just reflected in surface opinions and behaviours of Canadians — it is also defined by values. These are deep, beneath-the-surface convictions that may or may not be consistent with attitudes and behaviours but that will, ultimately, drive them.

The use of the term "values" is widespread yet there is much confusion about what values are and how they assist in decision making. We understand values to refer to relatively stable cultural propositions about what is deemed to be good or bad by a society. The distinction between values and such closely related concepts such as attitudes, opinions and beliefs is not, however, always clear. The most basic distinction is that whereas values are features of society and not specific to any object or situation, attitudes are understood at the level of the individual and organized or oriented toward a particular object or situation. A belief is any simple proposition, conscious or unconscious; inferred from what a person says or does; whereas an opinion is a verbal expression of some belief, attitude or value.

. . . an individual's attitudes are the product of a unique configuration of values and strategic interests, and the relative prominence given to each.

Health and health care present a complex, often emotionally intense, subject. Thus, relevant values often operate intuitively rather than "top-of-mind". Most of us are not ethicists with an explicit, articulated value system that can be applied deductively to situations as needed. We do have ethical systems but, in a complex area like health care, applying values is more a process of feeling the way we confront and deal with particular situations.

How we apply values to forming an opinion about a particular policy issue depends on the level of engagement with the issue — the amount of time and effort spent thinking about it, perhaps discussing it with others, and the quality of information about the issue. An opinion formed with relatively little engagement or with poor information will be less stable in the long term than one formed under conditions of high engagement and good information.

Although values are relatively permanent features of the societal landscape, individuals will appropriate values to form their attitudes to a given issue. The particular attitudinal combination varies through time and reflects an uneasy mixture of images, beliefs, interests and values. But these attitudes are important in as much as they influence behaviour (e.g., participation, support, protest). In addition, values are not shared by all members of a social group and attitudes are mediated to a certain extent by strategic interests. As a result, an individual's attitudes are the product of a unique configuration of values and strategic interests, and the relative prominence given to each.

What does this mean for policy development and acceptance of social policy? To the degree governments can impart good information, and provide mechanisms and incentives for citizens to think seriously about the issues, they will receive input to policy with a substantially longer and more predictable life span.

The role of knowledge in the development of attitudes was not fully explored in our research. Risk perception is largely a product of familiarity, knowledge and sense of personal control. For most Canadians, the potential for risk perception is very high since these factors are low in some policy areas. Yet it is not objective, but rather perceived reality which forms the challenge for delivering a new policy.

What are the connections between Canadians' core values and the health care system, and, more important, what are the implications for decisions and decision making? We explored these questions through some original public opinion research, using a series of scenarios or short stories which addressed many of the issues being investigated by the other working groups of the Forum. These scenarios, (see Appendix A) which illustrated the difficult choices currently being faced in the health system, were first screened as to form and content with a number of key informants who assisted the work of the Values working group. The scenarios were tested using the focus group methodology (see Appendix B). Participants were asked to make choices which showed a preference for certain values. Quantitative research supplemented the focus groups in order to enhance the generalizability of the findings. We also supported a review of public opinion research on health and social policy. Finally, we commissioned a review of Canadian and international experience with ethics bodies, to identify the contribution that such groups can make to continuing the discussion of values and decisions. In the following sections, key findings are outlined.

Key Findings

The findings have been clustered into common themes and issues. By simplifying the findings, we intend to identify the common values which emerged from the research. Moreover, as the qualitative portion of the data depended on eight scenarios presented to the focus groups, this section is more meaningful when read in conjunction with the scenarios and related questions.

Canadians value their health system

Throughout our work, we identified a number of values as central to most people's view of the health system. Our research revealed an interaction of strong vested interests and powerful values (pride, equality, compassion, national identity) which provides the capacity for rigorous debate in the future. At a time when other traditional expressions of Canadian values have been placed under demonstrable stress, health and health care have increased in importance and prominence as a shared and common value. In fact the health system has always engendered strong support among Canadians. In recent years, however, its significance has broadened into symbolic terms as a defining national characteristic.

At a time when other traditional expressions of Canadian values have been placed under demonstrable stress, health and health care have increased in importance and prominence as a shared and common value.

The values that the public continues to support can be grouped around several core themes.

Equality (or fairness)

Equality of access was one of the most important values consistently advocated. Canadians should have equal opportunity to achieve health and well-being and to receive health services according to their needs. The health care system allows all of us to share in the costs of health care on the basis of our ability to pay, through income and other taxes. The system is equitable and simple and reinforces an abiding sense of the fairness of equality in opportunity.

Compassion

The common good is of necessity the common concern. Organized effort in the control of health care is due to a desire to protect the strong as well as the weak and a recognition of our mutual dependency. Social solidarity and concern for the specially vulnerable also exist within the concept of the common good.

Dignity and Respect

Individuals are to be treated with dignity and their innate self-worth, intelligence and capacity of choice are respected.

Efficiency/Effectiveness

Due to the scarcity of resources, it is very important that health services be delivered in the most efficient fashion possible. The health system should achieve desired outcomes with the least expenditure, thereby providing good value for money spent. Efficiency has two important dimensions: minimizing the cost of the services provided and choosing those services leading to maximum benefits over costs. Waste and duplication are to be eliminated.

Collective Responsibility

People want to participate meaningfully in decisions about their own health system. Representation on community or regional boards and participation in community needs assessments are two forms of participation. Greater public involvement at a community level will ensure that needs and values of different cultural, linguistic and religious groups will be represented and upheld. Public participation is facilitated when sound accurate information is readily available, to ensure the system is accountable.

Personal Responsibility

Personal or individual responsibility has been, and continues to be, important to individual and population health and to the use of the health care system. Personal responsibility does not, however, translate into denial of medical coverage for personal choices which have an adverse impact on health. Such responsibility is overridden by the number one value — access to quality health care for all.

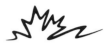

Quality

People want as high a quality of life and health care as possible. Quality of care and equality of access were frequently cited as the twin pillars of our health system.

Thriftiness — Responsible Stewardship — Accountability

Accountability is a necessary element of our socially-oriented health system and seen as having two current complementary needs: the need to encourage and educate Canadians toward increased responsibility for health, and the need for increased responsibility in the provision of health care services that meet public needs effectively and efficiently.

We found in our work that these values are deeply held and form a solid and stable foundation for public policy. Many have remained unchanged over time. What has changed, however, is the degree of certainty that Canadians have about the future of the health system. People are proud of the existing system and see it as a source of collective values and identity. They worry about the future viability of the system and are resistant to many of the alternatives currently on the table. Cynicism about change is high and the public rejects many of the premises for "reform". They believe cost problems are rooted in mismanagement and abuse, and would prefer to see these issues dealt with first. This being said, people still prefer using new public resources to preserve the integrity and core values of the system.

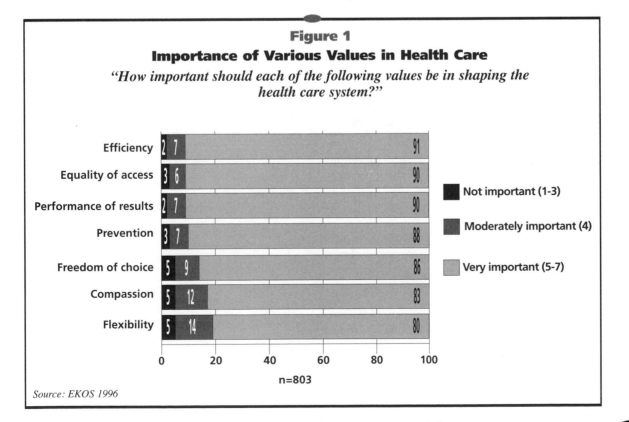

Figure 1
Importance of Various Values in Health Care
"How important should each of the following values be in shaping the health care system?"

Legend:
- Not important (1-3)
- Moderately important (4)
- Very important (5-7)

Value	Not important (1-3)	Moderately important (4)	Very important (5-7)
Efficiency	2	7	91
Equality of access	3	6	90
Performance of results	2	7	90
Prevention	3	7	88
Freedom of choice	5	9	86
Compassion	5	12	83
Flexibility	5	14	80

n=803

Source: EKOS 1996

In the quantitative portion of our research, participants were presented with a specific list of values and asked the relative importance of each in shaping health reform. The results which follow were combined with the results of the qualitative research and the findings from our national consultation process. This partly explains why the list of values in figure 1 differs in part from the preceding core values.

Many see "health reform" as a code for withdrawal of services and, consequently, there is concern about the viability of the system in the future.

As Figure 1 indicates, all values are believed to be important in shaping the health care system. However, efficiency, performance and equality of access are assigned highest priority. People also told us that the health care system had a special importance to them as Canadians: "...it's a basic fundamental tenent of being Canadian." Many agreed that the universality of the system helped distinguish Canada from the United States in a way that showed us to be a more generous and compassionate society. Others said that they derived a sense of pride with the quality of the system.

People feel they are very fortunate to have benefited from such a good system. Accessibility and quality are described as the twin pillars of the health care system, with accessibility being somewhat more important for the majority. We take pride that both rich and poor have access to the same quality of health services in Canada.

Our research required participants in focus groups to face trade-offs and choices which often shook their core beliefs and forced them to reassess long-held attitudes. Indeed, the majority of participants were ingenious at avoiding the hard choices. They see our health system as threatened but are loath to trade off the current system against the promise of a better or fairer future performance. Many see "health reform" as a code for withdrawal of services and, consequently, there is concern about the viability of the system in the future. Participants also expressed a desire for health care reform to reflect the values they believe in and to be undertaken with an eye to improving and preserving what they consider to be important about the system rather than just dismantling what exists.

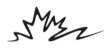

Concern for the Future

Many people told us of their concern that health care would not remain the same in the future. A significant number believed that health care in Canada was not as good as it had been because of government cuts in health care spending, longer waiting lists for doctors or procedures and the number of doctors leaving for the United States.

Regardless of whether they believed that the service had diminished already, almost all believed that the future of the system was threatened. High levels of government indebtedness have convinced most that greater cuts are likely in the future. That expectation is positioned against an under-standing that health care costs will continue to rise, especially for things like drugs and technology.

Some worried that the will to maintain the system was not strong enough, that there may be other ideological agendas at play, even undercutting the system. These people did not quarrel with the principle of governments getting their fiscal houses in order, but believed that some governments had agendas to diminish medicare by subterfuge — that the need for spending cuts provided cover to those who did not believe in the principles of the health care system.

When participants in our research spoke about the future of the system, almost all did so in bleak terms. Together, the participants' perception of the Canadian health care system in the 21st century was one of a system overburdened with aging baby boomers and "Americanized", complete with user fees and a growing gap between the level of care available to rich and poor. Few were opti-mistic that breakthroughs in health research, medical technology, public awareness about health issues or improved health care management systems would coalesce to counter some of the more ominous trends identified by participants.

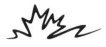

Canadian Pride and National Identity

The vast majority of those who participated in our research were immensely proud of the type of health care system that has been built in Canada. Almost all participants considered it to be strongly reflective of Canadian values and often contrasted it with the American system of health care.

Although other competing priorities emerged over the period of the discussions, *equality of access* is a primary one. The Canadian values are wrapped up in this equality — everybody gets relatively equal care when they are sick and nobody has to lose their house to pay their hospital or doctor bills. This is the feature which is seen to distinguish us most from the American model, which is the point of comparison.

Many people readily acknowledged that their commitment to egalitarianism is restricted to health care and that they are not troubled by wide discrepancies based on ability to pay or status in other areas of society. They have no trouble isolating health care in this way because they see it as something of a completely different character from housing or automobiles or vacations. It is also clear that many, perhaps most, believe that they, personally, might be worse off should the system evolve into two tiers.

One of the ways in which equality in health care is different stems from the fact that being as healthy as possible is seen to be fundamental to the quality of life that is part of being

Canadian. Most people fully accept that different income levels lead to different standards of living. However, most would not tolerate a situation in which one person does not receive the same treatment for a physical ailment as another on the basis of income. This form of inequality was unacceptable.

Equality of access is also seen to be essential to opportunity. Variances in income could be the end result of the market economy, but being physically healthy is seen as a precondition for having a fair chance at success. If there is to be equality of opportunity, then as far as possible everyone should start from a position of good health.

Finally, many saw our health system as a smart investment on the part of our country — one that gives us some comparative economic advantages and makes society more stable. At a time when the rapidity of change is proving deeply unsettling for many people and when economic change is having an adverse effect on many families, the fact that Canadians need not worry about either being unable to afford necessary medical treatment or being bankrupted by medical bills is seen as eminently sensible.

An overwhelming majority of participants stated that medicare was, and is, an essential part of their national identity. The different approach to health care is one of the main distinctions between Canada and the United States. In a period when the unity of the country is fragile and when people from coast to coast are struggling to find the common values and shared enterprise to keep the country together, it is perhaps both symbolic and disquieting that people perceive medicare to be threatened as this research suggests.

Canadian underpinnings of the health care system include the premise that it ought to be government run and not for profit, that money is not the primary consideration and that all are entitled — as a matter of citizenship — to equal access to quality care. This typically Canadian approach is, for many people, emblematic of a commitment to compassion, to equality of opportunity, to a sense of community and to a common purpose. However, this kind of approach is under attack every day from the forces driving change in society — high levels of government debt, globalization of the economy and the influence of international money markets.

Ultimately, the Canadian health care system, as it has operated for the last three decades, continues to enjoy broad and strong public support. In a period when belief in government efficacy is low, medicare is one government program that is popular and thought to be sensible. As popular at it is, people still understand it to be threatened. Nor are they are confused about what is threatening it. They understand it to be threatened by steadily rising costs and the inability of government finances to absorb those costs.

Participants in our research understand that change is coming — not out of desire, but of necessity. And for health care to retain its valued character, much else will have to change.

What the public wants from reform is a program that is consistent with the existing one: a high quality system founded on the principle that health care should be accessible, to all who need it, on an affordable basis. They like the way it works, the security and peace of mind that it provides. They like what is says about Canadians as a people.

Key Message:

The Canadian approach to the provision of health care services continues to receive strong and passionate support. The public does not want to see any significant changes which would alter the fundamental principles of our publicly administered health care system. They have an abiding sense of the values of fairness and equality and do not want to see a health system in which the rich are treated differently from the poor. The Forum supports this view and supports necessary changes to our health system only if we preserve the essence of medicare — universal coverage based on need, without financial barrier, portable across the country, to a comprehensive array of publicly administered health care services.

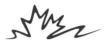

The Twin Pillars of Access and Quality

Our research found that equal numbers of people believed that equal access and quality of care were most important to them personally. Nothing else was of equivalent importance. People also tended to think that they reflected a consensus in Canadian society about values and health care.

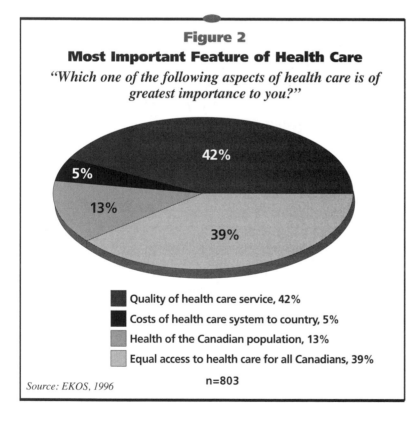

Figure 2

Most Important Feature of Health Care

"Which one of the following aspects of health care is of greatest importance to you?"

- Quality of health care service, 42%
- Costs of health care system to country, 5%
- Health of the Canadian population, 13%
- Equal access to health care for all Canadians, 39%

Source: EKOS, 1996 n=803

Our research showed that there is a consensus about the importance of equality of access as the defining characteristic of our system. That consensus is premised on the assumption that quality is a given, as people have perceived it to be in the past. However, if quality of service appears to be threatened, the consensus

over the importance of equality of access is much less firm. People believed that, historically, our health care had been better than, or at least equal to, anything in the world — with the possible exception of the care available to the very wealthiest Americans. Most thought that this was still the case, but that our system is threatened. Many were prepared to entertain significant changes in the way the system is designed and administered to preserve quality of care. There did not appear to be a similar willingness to accept significant reductions in the quality of care to preserve access.

Most participants demanded a very high standard of quality of care. Almost all seemed to accept that, in the world of endless technological advances and spiralling health care costs, not everything would be possible in our system. For example, most had no problem with the use of a less expensive heart drug in exchange for a minor increase in risk. But, on the other hand, participants volunteered concerns about a brain drain of doctors as evidence of their worries about the ability to maintain quality in our system with decreasing or insufficiently increasing dollars.

There are important assumptions built into the value choices that people make about health care. The debate about two-tier health care can be seen as a clash between individual and communal values. We found that most people feel free to place a higher priority on the communal values because quality and choice are seen as a given. Participants who opposed the introduction of a two-tiered system did so largely on the basis that no matter how private clinics were run and regulated and despite assurances which might be given about the preservation and preeminence of the public system, the core values of equality and fairness would suffer.

As a consequence, people are not choosing between competing values so much as they are layering communal values on top of a baseline expectation of service. This does not diminish communal values: they are strong and, given that they are not found in every country or society, the priority placed on them does speak to a Canadian values system. It is also true that, since Canadians recognize that a predominantly private system like the US version might provide even greater levels of quality or freedom of choice to at least some citizens, they are choosing to sacrifice some of that to provide equality of access to a universal system.

If convinced (and this constitutes a large "if") that governments could not afford to maintain the existing system, participants in our research were more comfortable with solutions that introduced more resources into the system to forestall a diminution in quality. For instance, some were willing to accept user fees for doctor or hospital visits, or to think that private clinics might be a way to get more money into the system. However, most did not advocate these as desirable approaches.

Key Message:

People want to ensure that our health system provides both equality of access and quality of care. There is also the impression, however, that there is a conflict between these two pillars of our health system and in order to have more of one you may have to give up some of the other. The Forum believes that this conflict is unfounded and that both equality of access and quality of care are not only possible but are readily achievable within our health system.

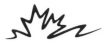

Support for Change that Increases Efficiency and Effectiveness

People generally agreed that the stress on the system was the result of fiscal pressures. Yet, most felt that these pressures resulted from mismanagement of the system (e.g., political expediency, poor administration, duplication, lack of planning, etc.) and from abuse and misuse of resources by patients and doctors. Other sources of fiscal pressure they cited included the rapid development of expensive medical technology and an ageing population. Recent reductions in health care budgets, and stories of their impacts, have made people somewhat less convinced of the extent of waste and abuse in the system. However, they want to see these problems addressed before contemplating other changes to medicare.

Recent reductions in health care budgets, and stories of their impacts, have made people somewhat less convinced of the extent of waste and abuse in the system. However, they want to see these problems addressed before contemplating other changes to medicare.

Abuse of the system was a main concern for all of our research groups, particularly seniors. People thought that some patients may be using the system fraudulently (e.g., non-residents receiving treatment with health insurance cards) but this was not the main concern. They believe the core problem is that too many people take the health care system for granted. Furthermore, overprescribing of drugs by physicians and the scheduling of unnecessary return visits were some of the other areas thought to require close attention and reform.

Most felt that patient misuse was not the result of wilful misconduct but rather due to ignorance about the workings and costs of the system and, more important, the result of poor judgment about appropriate courses of action to take in illness. Participants agreed that the population needed more information about these issues.

The general perception of most participants that fiscal pressures on the health care system were the result of mismanagement and abuse appears significant. Many believed that the alternative remedies of improving the management of the system and eliminating abuse and misuse had to be exhausted *before* some of the options described in the scenarios could be contemplated.

Participants in our research demonstrated a qualified acceptance of some form of user fee or alterative financing arrangement to deter these abuses. For one thing, alternatives would necessarily have to ensure that quality and access would not suffer. Some would willingly accept user fees for doctor or hospital visits. However, these same people did not want fees to be a deterrent for anyone in genuine medical need.

Some of those most concerned about fiscal issues ranked efficiency very highly. They were concerned that the absence of a cap on health care spending would have a negative impact on government deficits and tax rates. Most, however, did not want efficiency or cost concerns alone to be the driving force in health policy. Similarly, although virtually all participants were concerned about government deficits, they did not think that the health care system was the main problem. Most felt it was the highest priority and that savings should be found elsewhere.

Most people did believe that the maximum benefit for the dollar had to be a consideration for society. As discussed elsewhere, they did not like the trade-offs and did not confront them easily. However, there was a sense that health care dollars were not being spent most wisely. Combined with the belief that dollars were now very limited, this led to an acceptance by many that tough allocation decisions would have to be made to preserve the elements of real value in the system.

Key Message:

The public supports messages and measures which take visible action against perceived abuses and inefficiencies. In espousing the values of efficiency and effectiveness, there is an expectation that priority will be given to such measures before a consideration of other changes. The public want access to accurate information on proven effectiveness in order to provide them with better options to make educated consumption decisions. The Forum supports this view and supports the establishment of an information infrastructure accessible to both professionals and the public in order to meet this need.

Investing in Disease Prevention and Health Promotion

Most participants believed that the system ought to focus more on the broader determinants of health. The majority of participants were reluctant to shift resources away from direct health care to pay for programs aimed at promoting the general health of the population (e.g., job creation, cleaning up the environment). It is important to note here that a number of participants had difficulty following the counter argument in favour of channelling resources away from treatment toward improving the health of the general population. This difficulty may have been due to the fact that the positive correlation which exists between better health and higher levels of employment and education was not mentioned in the scenario.

Once participants understood the connection between improvements in the environment, education and other indicators of socioeconomic status, some supported a slight shift in funding aimed at promoting the general health of the population: "It makes sense. It's a long-term strategy about treating the cause rather than the symptom." Most participants were much less sanguine and remained reluctant to take funding away from health care to pay for "prevention programs at large," as one participant called it. Some said their opposition was mainly based on their inability to countenance a policy which would reduce health services, no matter how promising the long-term impact of a prevention strategy was. For others, opposition stemmed mainly from a lack of confidence in governments' ability to achieve the intended impact of health promotion and disease prevention programs (i.e., a healthier population).

Some participants in every group were strongly convinced of the merits of focusing on prevention and the root causes of health problems, including those caused by social and economic factors. Most participants had a more limited view of what constituted prevention; they confined it to the context of the health care system and tended to see it more along the lines of education about lifestyle or encouraging proper nutrition or fitness.

Most participants conceived of the health care system as an insurance policy for themselves and their family: they pay into it expecting one day to need it, and then have the right to draw on it and expect it to provide the required resources.

Some of the discussions brought into sharp focus the way in which participants think of health care and the health care system. Most drew a clear distinction between prevention issues that made great sense and would help to create a healthier population on one hand, and actual treatment, or what the health care system ought to concern itself with. Most participants conceived of the health care system as an insurance policy for themselves and their family: they pay into it expecting one day to need it, and then have the right to draw on it and expect it to provide the required resources. The fundamental responsibility of the health care system was seen to be treatment of the sick. Anything else is peripheral to its mission, including the reallocation of resources from treatment to prevention, because this might mean that they might not get the care they need.

Many thought that more emphasis on prevention could both provide a healthier population and result in long-term cost savings. Almost all older participants, and those who had indicated to the group that they had suffered a serious illness, supported this view. When forced to choose, participants saw prevention programs as intangible compared to the awesome and concrete nature of acute-care medicine. In addition, some participants expressed doubt about the effectiveness of prevention programs.

Support for health promotion and disease prevention measures, within the health care framework, is strongest when the measures are more tightly connected to traditional understandings of health care and are more limited and focused in scope. There was also a clear indication that some participants viewed prevention in terms of making healthy lifestyle choices which were largely a matter of personal responsibility. This view contributed to the resistance toward reallocating resources from prevention to treatment. Therefore, in addition to the lack of clarity as to what constituted prevention and promotion activities, there was a tendency among many participants to view prevention and promotion activities as being in competition with acute care. For many participants, it was fundamentally unacceptable to deny critical care because the resources had been spent on

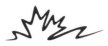

prevention. Indeed when prevention and promotion activities are viewed as being on a continuum with acute care, the confusion diminishes and the support for prevention and promotion becomes markedly pronounced. Research participants readily acknowledged that health is larger than health care and many of the determinants of health fall outside the health care sector.

Key Message:

The public strongly supports investment in disease and injury prevention and health promotion. They also strongly support a quality health care system. The Forum supports this view and believes that these are not contradictory goals but complementary to each other. We also support the view that the public needs more information and evidence on where promotion and prevention make a difference. Though there is an accountability factor in personal health choices, it should not be used to disenfranchise persons who need care.

The Expanding Spectrum of Health Care Services

The use of alternative and complementary medicines has increased exponentially in Canada in the last decade. Statistics Canada data indicate that over three million Canadians spent $1 billion in 1995 for alternative treatments not covered by traditional health plans.

In our research there was consensus among participants that the cost of alternative and complementary medicines and therapies, such as acupuncture and chiropractic procedures, should be covered by the health care system if they were proven to be effective. Such a pragmatic approach was largely based on the participants' generally positive personal experience with these therapies. However, most agreed that mere consumer demand did not constitute sufficient grounds on which to base a decision to use public funds for an alternative/complementary health service, treatment or medication. The notion that consumers (patients) should have an important say in the process appealed to participants, particularly in light of their perception that the medical establishment fought the inclusion of alternatives in the mainstream of the health care system. After some deliberation on the issue, however, there was general agreement that "scientific proof" or "medical evidence" was required before public funding of such a procedure.

In the end, there was agreement that enough consumer demand for an approach to be covered by the health care system should lead to objective study of its effectiveness. If it proved effective, the procedure should be covered, at least partially. To be considered effective, a practice or procedure must be proven to have a significant positive impact on patients. Moreover, an independent body or panel should be charged with the task of judging effectiveness.

Key Message:

As our research and consultations have shown, the public is not concerned about who provided the alternative or complementary medicine or therapy but rather whether or not it was effective. The public's acceptance of the integration of alternative and complementary medicines and therapies is therefore premised on the basis of proven 'effectiveness'. The Forum supports this view. If on the basis of the best evidence available the alternative or complementary medicines or therapies are effective then efforts should be taken to ensuring their availability. Conversely, if the available evidence indicates their harmfulness or ineffectiveness, the public should be protected.

Care Closer to the Home

Participants strongly agreed that it was not fair to expect families to assume increased responsibility for caring for their own members and that the state should not rely on such an assumption in making allocation decisions. They listed a number of mutually reinforcing arguments against even a slight shift of responsibility away from institutions and health care professionals toward families. The main objection was that such an approach ran counter to dominant societal trends, such as the growth of single parent families and families where both parents have to work, longer working hours, individualism, consumerism and atomization of society. Participants emphasized the significance of these trends as a way of showing that most people were not equipped, either financially or emotionally, to take on the sort of responsibilities described in the scenario. Other arguments against assuming responsibility included the following.

■ Parents have already been expected by the state to take on more responsibilities in other areas, such as the schooling of their children.

■ Older participants agreed that they did not want to burden their children and spouses. They also emphasized that it was naive to assume that they would even want to be taken care of by their children.

■ Younger participants echoed these views, with many frankly admitting that they simply could not handle the care of a parent.

■ Some expressed concern about the ability of a family member to care properly for a recovering patient, especially if the family member was older: "What if something goes wrong? Would we get training?"

The idea of compensating people who assume significant responsibility for looking after someone, through a tax credit for example, produced mixed responses. Some participants felt it was fair and reasonable. They supported a policy which would provide such compensation but which would not require anyone to assume more responsibility for a relative unless they freely chose to do so.

Others rejected the idea. A few said they found the idea of having the state pay people to take care of a relative distasteful. Others said that such a policy would open the door to abuse, particularly abuse of a parent. In the end, these participants preferred the state to stay away from the issue completely and leave matters to family members: "It has to come from the heart. People have to want to do it or else it won't work."

On balance there was considerable scepticism that government would put the required resources into the hands of people or communities. Many saw it as a thin veil for service reductions. On the other hand, participants also strongly agreed on a final point. They encouraged government to facilitate and fund home care and other forms of community-based care in which professionally trained personnel looked after people. For many research participants, it was their view that care in the home is not only cheaper but people recover faster and are happier in their own home. The qualification, however, was that professionals should look after people, not family members.

There was a strong consensus among the participants of our national consultations that the transition from institutional care to home care must be planned, managed and part of a comprehensive system of health care. Moreover, given that home care is multifaceted – ambulatory care, long term chronic care, palliative care, etc. – the planning must be tailored to the particular circumstances. Participants also highlighted the fact that home care is not an end in itself: it is a means to an end and it is only as good as the support available. Moreover, home care should be part of a continuum, well coordinated at the community level, using multi-disciplinary teams.

Key Message:

The public supports care in the home and other forms of community-based care but does not react well to being conscripted into care giving. Adequate and sustained government funding and the use of professionally trained personnel is a precondition for their support. The Forum supports this view. Shifting resources away from institutional care towards community-based services has been a common theme of health care reform in Canada and in many other industrialized countries. However, caregivers are fearful of being overwhelmed in the process. The Forum suggests that home care be defined as an integral part of the publicly funded health services.

On the other hand, participants also strongly agreed on a final point. They encouraged government to facilitate and fund home care and other forms of community-based care in which professionally trained personnel looked after people.

Ethical Reflection in Canada

As part of its exploration of values, the Values Working Group commissioned research which analysed the current structure and functioning of the various federal, provincial and regional ethics boards in Canada. Research has also been conducted into the structure and functioning of national ethics bodies in other countries to see whether the existing framework in Canada needs a more national centralized body for ethical reflection (Leroux et al., 1997).

It is clear from the research that Canada's approach to confronting ethical considerations can best be described as ad hoc.

It is clear from the research that Canada's approach to confronting ethical considerations can best be described as ad hoc. For instance, when faced with the ethical dilemmas emerging from the rapid development of new reproductive techniques, a royal commission was established; when confronted with the AIDS epidemic, the Federal Centre for AIDS was created; to investigate the legal problems surrounding assisted suicide and euthanasia, the Senate of Canada mandated a special committee to examine the issue. These of course, are not isolated examples, but serve as a testament to lack of a universal approach in addressing ethical issues.

This is not to say that there are not some quasi-stable mechanisms for addressing some of these issues. At the national level, we note that the Canadian Medical Association is the only body documented among Canadian professional associations to have a permanent ethics committee. Some of its member associations have created their own ethics committees. Other organizations such as the Canadian Nurses Association, choose to resolve ethical issues by means of particular committees. Research involving human subjects does receive more ongoing consideration with the involvement of such national bodies as the Medical Research Council of Canada and the National Council on Bioethics in Human Research.

In some nations, ethical reflection enjoys a more permanent, respected role in the operations of research and medicine. Where national ethics committees are in existence (Belgium, Australia, France, for example), all were established by either executive or legislative power. This institutionalization provides these bodies with legitimacy, not only in the medical/research arena, but also with the public. Of course, the legal, political and even cultural contexts which many of these nations offer, allow this legitimacy to exist.

Additionally, understanding the current and emerging importance of institutionalized processes for ethical reflection appears much more advanced in these nations. For example, the Australian Health Ethics Committee is mandated to carry out studies and to advise government on ethical, legal and social issues related to public health, medical practice and research on human beings, as well as to play a part in developing rules of conduct in the field of health. Clearly this demonstrates political willingness not only to create these bodies but also to engage in necessary discussion, which is central to their effectiveness.

Without question, a just-in-time method of creating specific working groups and committees to address ethical questions is not a sustainable method for ethical debate. There is a multitude of ethical dilemmas that face societies today — from debate on reproductive methods to implications on privacy posed by the advancing capability of information technologies. It is clear that the ad hoc approach cannot definitively answer these questions. It is also clear that the trend in other countries is towards national oversight bodies characterized by greater communication and coodination in which consensus is achieved on issues and solutions. However, none of the solutions found by other countries is ideal for Canada.

A viable direction for advancing ethical debate in Canada is that of strengthening the links between existing organizations and networks. As research commissioned by the working group notes, there is little, if any, communication and collaboration among ethics bodies at the local and provincial levels. There are no provincial federations of local ethics bodies and, save for Quebec and Alberta where institutional ethics networks exist, there is little evidence that the organizations communicate with each other. The obvious result is duplication of work, lack of information and resource sharing and, most important, the risk of not achieving global consensus on issues when one is necessary.

Encouraging permanent links where there were none before can be the first step in addressing fragmentation of efforts in the current ethical debate.

Key Message:

The Values Working Group has concluded that the present ad hoc approach in Canada of linking values with health policy issues is not acceptable. However, there were no obvious structural solutions in other countries which are ideal for Canada. We need to find a Canadian solution. As an inaugural step in the process of enhancing and improving ethical reflection in Canada, the federal Minister of Health should take the lead in discussing with his provincial /territorial counterparts and key groups with a substantial interest in ethics ways to establish permanent linkages among ethics networks and bodies.

An action plan to accomplish this objective should be developed. Moreover, Ministers should also consider the ways and means of involving the public in discussions of ethical problems related to health. Because decisions on these issues will undoubtedly address areas of life formerly considered private, the public will demand, and should be granted, the opportunity to be heard and considered as part of the decision-making process.

Conclusions

Health and health care has become top-of-mind for Canadians. It is something about which they care deeply and are very concerned, something in which they understand significant reforms are occurring and in which they believe dramatic changes will occur.

They want health care reform to reflect the values they believe in and want it to be undertaken with a view to improving and preserving what they consider to be important about it rather than dismantling what exists.

Health and health care are the dominant public policy concerns of most people in Canada. Our research reveals just how much thought participants had put into the issues under discussion. Relative to other research of this type, participants had fully thought through ideas and opinions. At the same time, the fact that research participants had given the issues considerable thought did not mean that their views were cast in stone. On the contrary, the difficulty of the trade-offs and choices that the scenarios forced on them required them to reassess long-held attitudes. Arguments put forward by some participants were often persuasive to others.

The research made the case very strongly that the debate over health and health care policy in this country exists in a very dynamic environment, one in which conflicting and powerful forces are at play. The debate itself has the potential to shape opinion.

We found that talking about issues of health and health care has a significant impact on attitudes and judgments. The most important influence was the simple process of sitting down and talking about these issues in a small group. A number of consequences resulted from discussion of the issues.

- People became more confident in the system — the sense of imminent decline of the current system was significantly lower after the discussions. This suggests that there are exaggerated fears about the system which can be calmed somewhat through dialogue.

- The importance of values increased and the role of costs and funding declined — this reflects a broader tendency for the groups to reject a purely economic analysis of health care issues. The evidence suggests that further dialogue will tilt the debate more toward the values end of the spectrum. Canadians want to participate and influence this crucial debate. Indeed, the public and experts do not share a common discourse about the public policy issues. As the research has also indicated, the public is ingenious at avoiding the hard choices. The public does not accept a purely economic analysis of the issues.

- The choices available should become more elucidated in the health reform debate. The exercise of choice requires extensive, accurate and timely information and education. This also entails access to publicly verified information on the performance of the health services. The public should have access to accurate information in order to make educated decisions.

- The Canadian perception of decreased equality of access and quality of care of our health services is, at least in part, due to perceptions of our inability to address areas of abuse and mismanagement within the system. Addressing these deficiencies should occur long before consideration of other approaches to health or health care.

- The Canadian public wants to ensure that the strong federal and provincial presence in health and health care continues. The consensus is that cooperation between the different levels of government is to be encouraged and conflict discouraged.

- The language surrounding the debate on two-tiered health care has become an obstacle to effective communication and has obfuscated many of the underlying issues. The real issue is a determination of what services should be funded by the public system and what services should be funded privately. The Forum recommends preserving existing publicly insured services.

- There is a need for a broader vision than that of the traditional curative medical care model. Canadians are interested in alternative and complementary approaches and want to know whether they are effective. The integration of alternative/complementary therapies on the basis of effectiveness should be encouraged and financially supported.

- The shift in recent years toward non-institutional care brings with it a number of consequences. Though Canadians are largely supportive of home care, they react strongly to being conscripted. The Forum recommends that home care be defined as an integral part of publicly funded health services.

- There can be little doubt that the issues surrounding the country's health care system have gained significant currency in recent years because they touch cherished and core values of Canadians. Health and health care are very much at the forefront for most people. A natural consequence of this interest and acuity is the need to involve the public further in health and health care decision making. Policy makers should continue to identify and incorporate values into the policy decision process. Qualitative and quantitative research should be used whenever possible, and policy options under consideration should be regularly provided to consumer groups, stakeholders and ordinary Canadians for their input and advice. Due consideration of the values held by Canadians will go a long way toward ensuring that the resulting policies are perceived as relevant and valid.

■ A more tangible means of accommodating
and incorporating values into the health and
health care decision making process can be
achieved by following the international
trend towards national oversight bodies.
Entrusted with examining issues of ethics
and values in health and health care, these
bodies are characterized by a greater degree
of communication, coordination and consensus than is presently the case in Canada.
The current state of affairs in Canada is ad
hoc and often results in piecemeal reflections on the problems of the day. Therefore,
it is recommended that the federal Minister
of Health take the lead in conjunction with
his provincial /territorial counterparts in
addressing this fragmentation and develop
means of managing the explosive growth in
ethical reflection. As a first step in this
process, we strongly recommend that existing organizations and networks be invited
by the Ministers to an inaugural meeting to
further develop an action plan. The research
data commissioned by the Values Working
Group would be of assistance to any such
initiative.

References

Ekos Research Associates Inc. and Earnscliffe Research and Communications. "Research on Canadian Values in Relation to Health and the Health Care System." *Papers Commissioned by the National Forum on Health*. Ottawa, 1997 (in press).

Exploring Canadian Values — Foundations for Well-Being. Canadian Policy Research Network, Study No. F-01, 1995.

Leroux L., S. Le Bris and B.M. Knoppers. "The Feasibility of a National Canadian Ethics Advisory Committee: Points to Consider." *Papers Commissioned by the National Forum on Health*. Ottawa, 1997 (in press).

Appendix A

SCENARIO 1

Although she tried to hide it, Charlie could see that his mother was in pain. The physiotherapy wasn't doing her any good. It had been almost a year since her back began troubling her, and nothing they had tried so far had helped. It was getting worse.

Mrs. Wong had come to live with her son Charlie and his family two years ago, after her husband died. It had been difficult for her to adjust to the way of life in their small, northern city. She missed Chinatown and her friends there, and all the comforts it provided her, especially since she had become sick.

When the first symptoms of her back problem appeared, Charlie's mother knew what it was at once. "I had this problem 10 years ago," she had told him. "I went to the Chinese healer and right away he could tell what was wrong. After four weeks of acupuncture, the pain was gone. But he told me it would probably come back again, and now it has."

There was no Chinese healer in the city in which Charlie lived, but there was a naturopath who practised acupuncture. He had a good reputation, but his treatments were not covered under the province's health insurance plan. Treatments didn't cost much—four weeks of treatment might cost about $500— but Charlie and his family didn't have that kind of money. They were having difficulty making ends meet as it was.

It was because of lack of money that Charlie had persuaded his mother to see his doctor almost a year ago, and after that another doctor, and then a physiotherapist.

It had gone on too long. Looking at his mother, he decided that in the morning, he would take his mother to the naturopath. And if the naturopath thought acupuncture would help, he would go to the bank and borrow the money.

It doesn't make any sense, he thought to himself. If my mother was in Chinatown, 600 miles away in the same province, the acupuncture treatments would be paid for because the Chinese healer belongs to a publicly funded clinic. Here in my city, the public system will pay much money for treatments that do not help her, but will not pay for the treatment that probably will.

QUESTIONS

1. Do you think the health care system should pay for acupuncture for Charlie's mother?

2. On what grounds do you think the system should decide which health services will be publicly funded? Evidence of effectiveness? Consumer demand for them? Medical opinion?

3 Western medicine is but one of many different healing methods developed over the years by different cultures. In a multi-cultural society, should we be more willing to embrace multi-cultural health care?

4. State whether, and why, you agree or disagree with the following statement: "The decision whether to fund a given health service should be based on evidence of effectiveness. If traditional cures and therapies from other cultures meet these standards, they should be funded. If not, they should not be."

5. Does fairness mean that different population groups, and in particular ethnic groups, have a right to an approximately equal share of money spent on them for health care?

SCENARIO 2

After waiting three weeks for an appointment, Mr. S., a 55-year-old independent truck driver, met with a heart specialist, who advised him he needed coronary bypass surgery. Unfortunately, it would take up to 10 weeks before he could have the surgery. Mr. S. was told that his angina was stable and not immediately life-threatening, but serious all the same. For his safety, and the safety of others, the specialist said he should not return to work and that she would review his fitness to work following the surgery.

Mr. S. complained that being laid up would bring him financial ruin and that it would be maddening to live under the shadow of the operation for that long. The doctor listened carefully and sympathetically, but responded that there was nothing she could do.

Dejected by this news, Mr. S. pulled some strings with an old friend and got a meeting with a specialist in another major city. That specialist said he could get him in for surgery in about two weeks.

Mr. S. was pleased about this, but curious about the reason for the difference in waiting lists between the two cities. He investigated, and discovered that five years earlier the regional board for the city in which he lives decided to spend more money on prevention and consequently to spend less on acute care.

The regional board in the other city, however, considered and rejected this option, and decided instead to ensure that programs like the coronary bypass program were well funded.

According to a recent newspaper article, the prevention program has been very successful. The incidence of heart disease in Mr. S's region has decreased by 5 percent and is a full 10 percent lower than in the region to which he travelled for the bypass. "Maybe the board in my region made the right decision," he remarked to his wife, "but I'm sure glad I won't have to suffer its negative consequences".

QUESTIONS

1. Given the information above, which Board do you think made the right decision, and why?

2. Is it consistent with equal access that there should be such great variation in waiting lists between different regions in the same province?

3. How would you rank the various criteria listed below for prioritizing people in a waiting list for a medical service? Are there any that you feel should definitely not be used and why?

    a) medical urgency
    b) benefit to the individual
    c) benefit to society
    d) age
    e) lifestyle factors
    f) first come, first served

4. Supposing there were a private clinic where Mr. S. could get quicker treatment:

a) Are private clinics delivering more timely health services to those able to pay for them inconsistent with the principle of equal access?

b) In deciding whether private clinics are a good or a bad thing, how much difference does it make whether they are in part subsidized by the government?

c) Is it unfair if people with money can get more timely or higher quality health care than people who have to rely on the public system?

5. How would you feel about the inequality that would exist in a two-tiered system in which the public system funded only the most basic and essential services and, a second, private system, delivered more "cadillac" services to those with the ability to pay?

6. How important do you think it is for people to have the freedom to purchase health care privately if they can afford to and believe that the add benefit is worth the cost?

7. If everyone's basic needs were met in the public system, but some people could get more timely treatment by paying for it privately, would this be a serious inequality? Would you be prepared to accept this inequality in order to allow those with means the freedom to spend their money as they wished?

8. How is health care different from other services in our society that are bought and sold in the marketplace? What, if anything, is so special about health care?

9. We tolerate many inequalities in Canadian society. Some people have big houses, other live in the street. Some people drive fancy cars, while others cannot afford to buy a car at all. Is inequality in health care different than in other areas of life? If so, why?

SCENARIO 3

Walking home from the community meeting, Mariella and Pablo continued the discussion about health care funding that had begun there.

Mariella: *I can't believe you supported the cuts to health care.*

Pablo: *It's not that I don't think health care is important. But I think we could get better value for our money-more health for our money-by spending this money on other things. That money would do a lot more good if we spent it on job creation and cleaning up the environment.*

Mariella: *I think it's much more important to look after the people who are sick right now than to improve the health of the general population. And besides, I doubt that the money saved would be spent on making a difference in health. Our health care system is one of the things that makes this country so special, Pablo, and I'm very worried about the impact of these cuts.*

Pablo: *You heard what the experts at the meeting said. There's lots of waste and inefficiency. If we get rid of that, there's plenty of money to fund the system.*

Mariella: *I'm not so trusting. Maybe there is lots of inefficiency, but do you really believe that quality won't suffer? These cuts will make it very difficult for the provinces to ensure that all Canadians have equal access to high quality, medically necessary care.*

Pablo: *That term "medically necessary" is so broad it can mean anything. The health care system has expanded beyond its original intent, and beyond what we can afford. Sure, we have to see that no Canadians will lose their houses or burden themselves with debt in order to meet their medical needs, but maybe the government just can't afford to meet all the lesser needs and wants.*

Mariella: *Well, who's going to decide what we can and cannot afford, and which and whose needs are greatest? People like the ones at the meeting who supported the cuts? Most of those people were very well dressed and pretty healthy looking. Not very typical of the people I work with every day in the chronic care unit. And not very typical of the people in the neighbourhood where you and I grew up Pablo. Those are the people I care most about.*

Pablo: *We agree then Mariella, because it's these people I care most about too. I want them to have jobs, and I want their children to have good schools and safe streets. Those things don't come from doctors and hospitals.*

QUESTIONS

1. Which of the two speakers do you most sympathize with, and why?

2. Mariella is concerned about the consequences of funding cuts for poor and needy people. How important is the government's obligation to help these people? Is there anything else more important?

3. State whether, and why, you agree or disagree with the following statement: "We can't afford to pay for everything the public wants; we have to concentrate on what the public really needs."

4. In deciding the level of public funding for health care, how much weight should be given to what patients or consumers would like as opposed to what experts think they need?

5. Do you believe that all Canadians have a right to health care, and if so, how would you qualify this right? A right to basic services? A right to quality services? A right to the best health services possible?

6. Mariella thinks our health care system has special importance for us as Canadians. Do you agree? What significance or value does our health care system have for you as a Canadian citizen? Is there anything else about this country that you think is more important?

7. Some people claim our health care system is vitally important to our national identity. Do you agree? What is it about our health care system that makes you most proud as a Canadian?

   a) its high level of quality
   b) its efficiency
   c) its success in meeting the needs of the sick and vulnerable
   d) its equality

SCENARIO 4

Jimmy was terribly sick, but Nurse J. could tell from the faint smile he formed as she entered the room that he was very happy to see her familiar face. Young Jimmy Brown, nine years old, was no stranger to her care. This was his third visit to the emergency department since the fall. She clutched his hand and said, "Everything will be all right now Jimmy. We'll look after you."

Jimmy Brown has chronic asthma, and his condition had deteriorated since his last visit. This time Nurse J. was very worried from the signs she saw. They would look after him and give him the best care possible, and probably he would get better. But everything wouldn't be all right. In a week or so, if everything went well, he would go home, but that wouldn't make everything all right. Far from it. That was where the cycle would begin again.

Since his father had abandoned him and his mother two years ago, Jimmy had lived in a dilapidated old house on the outskirts of town. And in that house—a shack others might call it—was a wood stove that served as the only source of heat. Jimmy's mother knew that the fumes from the smoke aggravated his asthma, but there was nothing she could do. She didn't have the money to buy a furnace or to move into a better place. And the welfare system wouldn't cover it. Nurse J. and the social worker had tried their best to intervene on the Browns' behalf, but to no avail.

Nurse J. felt frustrated and angry. The system could not or would not do anything to remedy the problem that was causing Jimmy's sickness, but whenever he got really sick the system would go into high gear and spend many times more money that the cost of a furnace to fix him up. And the cycle would begin again.

It didn't make sense: not for Jimmy, not for his mother, and not for society. They wouldn't look after him, not really. It wouldn't be all right. It was only February, and there were cold months ahead.

QUESTIONS

1. Would it be appropriate to redirect money from sickness care to prevention if the money spent on prevention would produce more benefit, and perhaps even save money in the long run?

2. Do you think it is more important to ensure that people who are sick and disabled are able to achieve the best level of health possible or to ensure that people who are healthy do not become sick and disabled?

3. If the same amount of money could be used either to save the lives of 10 heart attack victims over a 5 year period, or through preventive measures to reduce the number of people who would suffer heart attacks over the same time period and thereby save 100 lives, which would you choose? Why?

4. In some cases, the cost of treating someone who is sick and in need are very great, and the anticipated benefit is uncertain and slight at best. In other cases however, tremendous benefits can be had for very little cost. If you had to choose between producing very slight benefit for one very sick person, and a greater benefit for 10 people who were less sick, which would you choose, and why?

SCENARIO 5

The newly formed Springdale Regional Board is responsible for health services, including hospitals and chronic care facilities, for a community of 300,000 people.

Each year, the Board receives a fixed sum of money from the province, which it must divide among health institutions, agencies and services in its region. Money is tight , and the Board has learned that it must make do with 10 per cent less money than it got last year. It has ordered an extensive review of all services to assist them in setting priorities.

The study disclosed that many health needs were not being adequately met by existing services. The needs of people who were dying were identified as an area of special concern, especially in light of the region's mission to ensure that people who chose to do so will be able to have a good death in the personal environment of their homes rather than in institutions. The study found that, overall, very little money was spent on palliative care compared to other health services and to acute care in particular. The report concluded, "We spend a tremendous amount of money trying to save lives even in cases where the chances of success are very slight. Money is no object here, it seems. But once it is decided that further aggressive treatment is futile or undesirable, we turn our backs on the dying and spend very little money to ensure that they have as good a death as possible."

Board members agreed that the needs of the dying were not being adequately met and agreed also about ways to improve the situation. However, these strategies require additional money, and, given the cuts to their bud-

get, there wasn't even sufficient money to fund existing programs. "The bottom line is that we cannot go on leaving these needs unmet," one member said. "We have to find the money to do this, and regrettably this will mean shifting it from other services. A good part of our budget goes to acute care, and I see little choice but to reallocate some money from acute care to palliative care. Given the other demands on our resources, maybe we can't afford that heart-lung transplant program at the main hospital. Very few people benefit from it, and the money could accomplish a lot more good if we spent it on the dying."

QUESTIONS

1. How important do you think it is to ensure that the needs of the dying are met as fully as possible compared to trying to save lives when chances of success are very poor?

2. Interventions to save lives are often very expensive. Do you think we put too much emphasis on saving lives at any cost at the expense of not meeting other important needs?

3. If we cannot afford to meet all heath care needs, on what grounds should we decide which needs will receive greater priority?

4. Is the amount of benefit produced per cost an appropriate criteria for deciding which, whether, and at what level health services should be funded? What alternative criteria would you suggest, and how would you compare their importance?

5. If two services are compared in terms of how much benefit each produces in terms of cost, and both cannot be funded, should

we fund the one with greater benefits per cost?

6. In deciding where to allocate health care resources, how important is it to you that the benefits are distributed fairly among various populations? How important is this consideration compared to ensuring that the greatest amount of benefit possible is produced, regardless of who gets what and how much of it?

7. How does information about how much money per person is spent on people in different groups bear, if at all, on fairness?

8. If you had to choose between funding a service that delivered three healthy meals a week to shut-ins, needy seniors, and a school lunch programme that provided lunches for needy children, which would you choose? Why?

9. What does fairness mean to you, and how important do you think it is for health care resources to be distributed fairly? How do you see the relationship between fairness and equality?

SCENARIO 6

"It's hard to say at this time how serious the heart attack was", the younger doctor said. "I think she'll be fine with the streptokinase."

"Let's hope so", the older doctor replied. "I'm not happy with the new guideline. If this happened a week ago, we would have used TPA, and I would have felt better about that."

The doctors must not have realized that the woman in the elevator with them was Mary S., the daughter of the 62-year-old woman they were talking about. Mary had eaves-dropped intently on their conversation, but hesitated to identify herself and ask the questions that were burning in her mind. She had decided instead to return to the floor and ask the nurse. The answers she received troubled her.

The nurse explained that there are currently two drugs available for treating heart attacks: streptokinase and r-TPA (tissue plasminogen activating factor). R-TPA is slightly more effective in severe heart attacks. Some research shows that it saves about one additional life for every 100 uses. However, the cost difference between the two drugs is great. Whereas streptokinase costs $460 per dose, r-TPA costs $2,500 per dose, more than five times as much.

The costs of a policy of using r-TPA in every case would be enormous, the nurse explained. Given budget constraints, the hospital pharmacy had recently examined its policy in this area and debated whether the benefit, in terms of the number of lives saved, was worth the costs. This money, it was claimed, could be used to better effect in the hospital. Some people thought the hospital pharmacy shouldn't carry it, but that doctors would only use it when they thought the heart attack was very severe. That was probably the guideline Mary heard the doctors talking about, the nurse figured.

Mary went back into her mother's room. She was sleeping now, and her vital signs were looking good. She was a strong woman, Mary thought. She'll be home and back out in her beloved garden in no time at all, Still, it troubled her to think that her mother might not have received the best treatment possible.

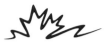

QUESTIONS

1. Suppose the money saved from this guideline could be used to achieve greater benefit (save more lives) in the hospital by being allocated in other ways. Do you think it is acceptable to use the cheaper but slightly less effective drug? Why?

2. Suppose that the money saved by using the cheaper drug was enough to fund a nurse to offer low-income families prenatal care in their homes, and that more lives could be saved by such a programme than by always using the more expensive drug. If you had to choose between these options, which would you choose, and why?

3. If the more expensive treatment slightly increased patient comfort, but would have no long term impact on the patient's health, do you think it should be offered, even though the benefit for this additional cost would be relatively small compared to other uses to which the money could be put?

4. All of us want the best care possible for ourselves and our loved ones. We also want to ensure that there is enough to go around, and that everybody gets a fair share. Do you think these two wants are ever in conflict? If so, how would you resolve the conflict?

5. Should we always do what is best for the individual patient, regardless of costs, or should we try to ensure that scarce health care dollars are used to produce as much benefit as possible?

6. Do you feel that the doctors have compromised their professional ethic by using the arguably second best treatment?

7. If a physician is aware of a treatment that would be more beneficial for you than any he or she is able to offer, is he or she obliged to disclose this information to you?

8. Should physicians ever by put in a position where they are required to do anything less than what they believe is in the best interests of their patients?

SCENARIO 7

There was a profound sadness in the cafeteria. After months of rumours, it was final now. The hospital would be closing.

"They say this community doesn't need two hospitals," Nurse L. remarked. "We're bursting at the seams with more people than we can look after, but the hospital isn't needed? Obviously we're meeting somebody's needs. How will those needs be met when we close? I don't get it."

"Oh, I get all right," Nurse S. said. "That's where community-based care comes in. These needs will be met in the community, closer to home. You know, self-help and all that, families taking more responsibility to look after their own. That's the story the public is expected to buy, hook, line and sinker."

"I think you're being a little too cynical," Nurse J. broke in. "Community-based care makes a lot of sense. You know as well as I do that many of the people we care for could just as well be cared for in the community or in their homes."

"Oh, I agree that a lot of them could be," Nurse S. replied, "if there were a community support system, or a family able to look after them. But the reality is that in too many cases there just isn't. And until there is, it's

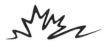

not right to dump sick people into the community."

"I agree," Nurse L. joined in. "And it's not just the patients I'm concerned about, it's their families—the mothers, sisters and daughters—who will bear the burden of caring for their needs. Undoubtedly this hospital isn't the best place for elderly people like Mr. J. in room 312. Nothing we can do will cure old age. But there's nowhere else for him to go except home, and then the burden of care will fall on Mrs. J. At her age it would be too much for her. Next thing you know, she'd be the one in the hospital. Community-based care—I'm all for it, if the community supports are in place. They say they're going to transfer some of the money saved from closing the hospital to the community and build up the support system. Why don't they do that first?"

"I'll tell you why," Nurse S. volunteered. "Because they have no intention of building up the support system, that's why. We've seen all of this before. Saving money is the name of the game here, and community-based care is just a smokescreen."

QUESTIONS

1. Do you think it is fair to expect families to assume increased responsibility for caring for their own? Is it fair to rely on such an expectation in making allocation decisions?

2. In some cultures there is a greater expectation that families will look after their own than in others. Is such an expectation something that we should try to foster more widely in our society?

3. When the burden of caring for someone is transferred from an institution to a family, should some part of the money thus saved be transferred to the family to assist them?

4. If costs can be saved by relying less on professional care-givers and more on family members and informal care groups, is it justifiable to pass this burden onto them? On what grounds?

5. Should charities and volunteers be expected to assume more of the burden of care presently being delivered in institutions or by the publicly-funded health care system?

SCENARIO 8

Joe was feeling a little nervous. As a respected leader in his community, he had been asked by the Regional Health Board to hold a meeting with his people to gauge their values about priorities for health spending in the region. He examined the list of values they had prepared for him to go over at the meeting:

Efficiency: The health system should be as efficient as possible. Services and programs should be effective, used appropriately and delivered at the least cost possible.

Comprehensiveness: The range of services should include all treatments and services that meet health needs.

Quality of care: The quality of care available to all Canadians should be as good as, or better than, what is available in other countries.

Patient autonomy: Patients should have maximum choice in deciding what services and treatments are available to them, and under what terms they will receive them.

Equal access for individuals: Every Canadian should have equal access to health care. Ability to pay should not be a barrier.

Equal shares for groups: Resources should be distributed such that different communities and population groups get equal shares.

Neediest first: Resources should be distributed on the basis of need: the needs of the neediest should be met before or ahead of the needs of the less needy; resources should be distributed to individuals and populations in proportion to their need for them.

Maximum benefit for dollar: We should strive to get the most "bang for buck" or benefit for the health care dollar.

A healthy population: We should strive to make as great a positive impact on the health and well-being of the Canadian population as possible.

Important issues were at stake. The budget for the Health Board had been cut back, and there were some difficult choices to be made. His community would be affected. He thought it was important that these choices be based on values instead of politics, and that the Board was wise to try to gauge the values of the communities it represented. Even so, values are hard to capture, and Joe wondered how well the values on the list captured the values of people in his community and whether the meeting would succeed in bringing their values to the surface.

QUESTIONS

1. How would you rank the principles listed above, and why? Are there any values you think should be added to the list?

2. What conflicts do you see as potentially developing among or between these values, and how would you resolve them?

3. Do you think most Canadians share the same values about health care and health care funding, or do you think there is a lot of variation based on things like cultural and religious differences? If different cultures do have different value priorities, how important do you think it is for the health system to reflect those differences?

4. Should people from different cultures be able to decide how and by what means their health needs will be met, or should health care services be the same for everyone?

Appendix B

Methodology: Qualitative and Quantitative Research

A core group of questions were used to initiate the discussion in all of the focus groups. These initial questions allowed participants a chance to begin thinking about the broader issues of values and health and the health care system and to provide spontaneous reflections on the study issues before the scenarios were presented.

Participants' views about underlying values were obtained by using eight "scenarios" (Appendix A) designed to highlight one or two key issues. The eight scenarios were selected by the research team, in consultation with the National Forum on Health, from 12 scenarios designed by the Forum. The eight chosen were those which the research team felt would be the most appropriate for use in the group discussions. While the scenarios were tested across all the focus groups, only two were discussed in any one particular group. This ensured that each scenario and its accompanying questions received adequate time for processing and reflection by focus group participants. Each scenario was tested in four different groups.

Participants were provided with a text version of the scenario and an audio-tape version. Participants were able to follow the scenario using their written version as the tape was played. The inclusion of the audio-tape version made it easier for participants to digest the content of the scenarios.

In 10 of the 18 focus groups, a "deliberative" exercise was conducted. This involved providing participants with some basic factual information about the Canadian health care system . The moderator walked participants through six graphs and solicited their reaction to the material. The purpose of the deliberative segment of the groups, which lasted 10 to 15 minutes, was to assess whether or not providing participants with information had an impact on their views. Impact was measured in terms of participants' subsequent comments in the groups, as well as by comparing their responses to the pre- and post-surveys. (The findings from the deliberative excercise can be found in the primary research document, *Research on Canadian Values in Relation to Health and the Health Care System*, Ekos Research Associates Inc. and Earnscliffe Research and Communications.

Focus group participants were drawn randomly from the general public. Using a script, recruiters introduced the study to the people contacted, applied the screening criteria and invited those who met the criteria to participate in the study. A total of 145 people participated in the focus groups; there was an average of approximately eight participants per focus group.

The quantitative survey portion of the research utilized potential participants contacted during the focus group recruitment stage. Potential participants were screened using a four-minute, 14-item questionnaire examining attitudes concerning the study issues as well as general demographic characteristics. After the potential participants had completed this battery of questions, they were asked if they would be willing to participate in a focus group session. A total of 800 individuals were asked this battery of questions.

Post-Participation Questionnaire: At the conclusion of each focus group session, participants were asked to respond to another short attitudinal questionnaire, which encompassed the same set of questions as the screening questionnaire.

The quantitative component yielded the following two data outputs: a 14 item survey of 803 people living in and around the nine centres in which the focus groups were conducted, and 93 matched pre-and post-surveys of focus group participants.

The design of the research aimed to include the participation of a cross-section of Canadians. Additional details on the selection criteria are presented below.

EXHIBIT 2.1
Language and Composition of Focus Groups

Location	Group Type	Deliberative Exercise
Ottawa (2) (pilot)	General population (25-60 years)	
	General population (25-60 years)	✔
Halifax (2)	Activists (25-60 years)	✔
	General population (25-60 years)	
Montreal (2)	General population (60+ years)	
	General population (25-60 years)	
Quebec City (2)	Activists (25-60 years)	✔
	General population (25-60 years)	
Windsor (2)	Activists (25-60 years)	✔
	General population (25-60 years)	✔
Sudbury (2)	General population (60+ years)	✔
	General population (25-60 years)	✔
Regina (2)	General population (Aboriginal)	
	General population (25-60 years)	✔
Edmonton (2)	Activist (25-60 years)	✔
	General population (25-60 years)	
Vancouver (2)	Activists (60+ years)	
	General population (25-60 years)	✔
TOTAL	**18 focus groups**	**10 deliberative exercises**

- *Centre Size:* Both large cities (e.g., Vancouver, Toronto, Montreal), as well as smaller centres (e.g., Regina, Quebec City, Sudbury) were selected as it was anticipated that residents from smaller centres may have different views/concerns about the health care system.

- *Age:* 1) People under 25 years of age were excluded because they were expected to be somewhat detached from the issue of the health care system and, thus, would be less involved participants in the groups.
2) Four groups with individuals aged 60 years and up were formed to ensure that the particular views of this important segment of the population, especially in the context of health and the health care system, were collected in the research.

- *Language:* Four groups (in Quebec) were conducted in French with the remaining groups being conducted in English.

- *Activism:* We conducted four groups with a subset of the Canadian population who are more involved in current issues as past research has demonstrated that this third of Canadians tend to have a significant influence on public policy debates.

- *Aboriginal Canadians:* A focus group with Aboriginal Peoples from the Regina area was conducted.

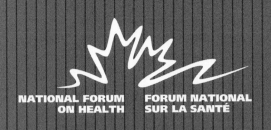

Striking
a Balance
Working
Group
Synthesis
Report

Striking a Balance Working Group

Steven Lewis (Chair)
William R.C. Blundell, B.A.Sc.
Richard Cashin, LL.B.
André-Pierre Contandriopoulos, Ph.D.
Robert G. Evans, Ph.D.
Tom W. Noseworthy, M.D.

Marcel Saulnier (Policy Analyst)

Contents

Introduction 3

Health Reform in Canada and Abroad 4

　Provincial reviews and reforms 4

　Developments at the national level 6

　An international perspective 7

Three Key Dimensions of Balance 9

　The balance between the health sector and the rest of the economy 11

　The balance of services within the health sector 13

　The public/private balance within the health sector 14

Rebalancing at the Societal Level 17

　A clearer mission for Canada's health system 17

　Are we spending too much or too little on health care? 19

Rebalancing Within the Health Sector 23

　Shifting toward non-institutional care 23

　Health system organization — in search of the magic bullet 26

The Public/Private Balance Within the Health Sector 34

　Reinforcing the role of public financing 34

　Improving access to health services 37

　Defining medically necessary services: holy grail or red herring? 40

Conclusion 44

Endnotes 45

References 46

Introduction

The Working Group on Striking a Balance was given the mandate by the National Forum on Health to examine how to allocate society's limited resources to best protect, restore and promote the health of Canadians. Attention was to be given to the balance of resources within the health sector as well as between the health sector and other sectors of the economy.

The impetus for this mandate came from a number of sources.

- First, there were concerns among Forum members that our health care system was consuming an ever increasing share of society's resources at a time when emerging knowledge on the determinants of health suggests that spending more on health care is not enough to improve health.

- Second, there were concerns that shifts within the health sector which have been advocated for years — from treatment to prevention, and from institutional to community-based services — have been implemented without the appropriate evidence to guide the pace of change.

- Third, there were concerns that the balance between public and private financing for health care was shifting by accident, rather than by design, thereby threatening nation-wide entitlement to universal access to health care based on need, which could well have profound health implications in the longer term.

Over the last 18 months, the Working Group on Striking a Balance commissioned a number of papers to generate insight in response to these concerns (see references appended). We conducted a thorough review of international trends in health expenditures, use of resources and outcomes. We devoted considerable attention to public and private financing issues, health system organization and federal-provincial transfers. We also produced a separate discussion paper on public and private financing which was widely circulated, and a position paper on the Canada Health and Social Transfer (CHST) which was endorsed by the Forum and submitted to the federal government.

Via the Forum's broader consultation process, the Working Group sought the views of the public and stakeholders on several issues germane to our mandate. Their valuable contribution has enriched and expanded our own thinking. We have also addressed several issues jointly with other Forum Working Groups, in particular the Determinants of Health Group and the Evidence-Based Decision Making Group. The outcome of our discussions with the Evidence-Based Decision Making Group on pharmaceuticals, given its scope and implications, is the subject of a separate report. (NFOH, Directions for a Pharmaceutical Policy, 1997)

Our objective in this report is to go beyond a simple restatement of health reform rhetoric. There are some real issues to be confronted if we are serious about striking a balance to improve the health of the public and to strengthen medicare. We now know in which direction public policy needs to change to improve population health. However, as a society, we have yet to find the political structures and mechanisms, the public support and the policy instruments necessary for this rebalancing to occur. At the same time, we must be careful about advocating for change within and outside the health sector which could be detrimental to the health care system and its capacity to deliver high quality health care based on need, not on ability to pay.

In the following pages, we review the key lessons learned from recent health reform efforts across the country and abroad. Next, we discuss the three key dimensions of balance which are most important from a health and health care perspective. We then delve into a number of issues specific to each of the three dimensions of balance. Each major section ends with a set of recommendations.

Health Reform in Canada and Abroad

The history of health policy in the industrialized world during the 20th century has been characterized first by the rise of conventional medicine and the sickness insurance movement, followed by increased attempts at controlling health care costs and a search for alternative pathways to health improvement (Evans, Barer and Marmor, 1994). Over the last few years, significant reforms have occurred in all provinces and at the national level. Abroad, virtually all industrialized countries have taken major steps to revamp their health care systems. As a backdrop to the more substantive discussion which follows, we report here on the most salient aspects of provincial, national and international reforms as they relate to our mandate.

Provincial reviews and reforms

It is often said that the last few years have seen a period of unprecedented change in the health sector in Canada. However, it is the *direction* rather than the *magnitude* of change that is truly unprecedented. It is true that from the late 1950s to the early 1970s, the system expanded considerably after the adoption of universal hospital and medical insurance across the country. During the 1970s and early 1980s, it further expanded as provinces implemented new programs and services beyond those under the federal-provincial cost-sharing arrangements. Starting in the mid-1980s, however, provinces felt a need to conduct extensive reviews of their health systems. This was the beginning of a different kind of change.

That something of the magnitude of a royal commission or task force is needed to have a comprehensive look at such a large and complex sector is to be expected. That seven of 10 provinces undertook such a review within a period of five years, however, suggests something more.[1] Not surprisingly, a number of common themes and initiatives have emerged from these reviews. We have incorporated these into our thinking. While it is not the intent of the Working Group to examine these in any detail, we do provide a status report on reforms and their links with our work.

First, without exception, all reviews have concluded that the health care system needs better management, not more money. We believe this to be true today, even though health care budgets have been frozen or reduced in many jurisdictions over the last few years. That is not to say that reductions in funding have no effect on access and choice of intervention. But reductions necessarily adversely affect quality only when the system is 100 percent efficient, or when spending is precariously low to begin with. This is far from self evident given that we spend roughly $2,500 per capita (of which $1,800 is publicly funded) or just under 10 percent of GDP on our health care system.

Second, although much has been written and said about the need to broaden the definition of health at the level of society and to shift the emphasis of the health care system toward prevention, efforts to date have met with limited success. Reasons for this may include: public attitudes and expectations; fiscal restraint; political cycles which make

long-term investments difficult to initiate and sustain; stove-pipe machinery of government which discourages intersectoral collaboration; entrenched stakeholder interests; inadequate research and evaluation, etc. More on this later.

Third, although provinces have made significant changes in the organization and delivery of health care, incentives need to be realigned if the efficiency and effectiveness of the system are to be further improved while maintaining universal access. This will require funding streams and decision-making structures to become more integrated, more focussed on outcomes and more centred on the patient/consumer.

. . . it is essential to maintain public confidence in the system throughout this continuing period of retrenchment and experimentation.

Finally, unlike previous waves of reforms which have been expansionary in nature, it is essential to maintain public confidence in the system throughout this continuing period of retrenchment and experimentation. Research by the Values Working Group has clearly shown that equal access to health services is highly valued by Canadians, though not at the expense of a significant deterioration in the quality of services. Mechanisms must be found to increase transparency and public accountability so that the public can judge the system's performance for themselves on an ongoing basis.

Developments at the national level

The latest sweep of provincial reforms has taken place within a very different environment at the national level than previous reforms. From the late 1940s to the early 1980s, the national environment was characterized by a number of expansionary and stabilizing forces, starting with federal hospital construction grants under the Health Resources Fund, followed by the *Hospital Insurance and Diagnostic Services Act* (1957), the *National Medical Care Insurance Act* (Medicare) (1966), the replacement of cost-sharing arrangements in 1977 with block funding under Established Programs Financing, and the *Canada Health Act* (1984). Over the last 10 years, however, rationalizing and potentially destabilizing forces have altered the national environment. These include extraordinary attention to cost control, the overall climate of fiscal restraint at both the federal and provincial levels, progressive reductions in federal transfer payments to provinces, as well as public policies such as the extension of patent protection for drugs. Whether these latter forces prove to be catalysts or irritants in the process of health reform depends on one's perspective.

Certainly, the emphasis placed on controlling health care costs was not without intellectual foundation. Starting with Lalonde's *A New Perspective on the Health of Canadians* (1974), Epp's *Achieving Health For All* (1986) and the *Ottawa Charter for Health Promotion* (1986), the emphasis for improving the health prospects of Canadians was increasingly placed on factors outside the health care system. This evolving analytical framework has been the backbone of national efforts to curb tobacco use, substance abuse, to encourage physical activity and to invest in a broad range of public health interventions. More recently, this thinking has been reframed to focus more directly on the root determinants of health — socioeconomic status, social supports, etc. — rather than on lifestyle issues. This has been at the heart of recent work by the Canadian Institute for Advanced Research, *Why are Some People Healthy and Others Not?* (1994) and the Federal/Provincial/Territorial report, *Strategies for Population Health* (1994).

It is not entirely clear where this line of thinking will lead, particularly given that action on the determinants of health — income distribution, employment and labour market policies, and early childhood development to name only a few — lie outside the ambit of the health sector. It does, however, suggest that the mission of the health sector will become even more complex. In addition to maintaining universal access to health care, more attention will be given to population health interventions within and outside the scope of the health sector. As we shall elaborate further, we must be clear about accountability for achieving healthy public policy, population health objectives and health care quality/access objectives — otherwise, the health sector will be increasingly burdened with responsibilities it cannot possibly fulfil, the superficial attractiveness of private care will become irresistible, and the tough political decisions needed to make a real difference in population health will be conveniently deferred.

An international perspective

Our review of international comparisons of resource allocation and outcomes suggests that industrialized countries face very similar challenges in maintaining universal access to quality health services while controlling costs.

Table 1 provides a snapshot of how Canada compares with OECD countries with respect to key health and health care indicators for 1994 (or the latest year available). On balance, and notwithstanding data compatibility issues across countries, Canada appears to have a relatively young and healthy population and a fairly well-developed, yet well-constrained, health care infrastructure. However, it has very high health expenditures. Further analysis of this data has revealed a number of interesting observations.

First, there are several ways to measure health expenditures, and each has its advantages and limitations. Accordingly, while Canada had the second highest ratio of health expenditures over GDP in 1994, our ranking slips to third place if we use per capita expenditures adjusted for purchasing power parity (PPP), and to 10th place if we use per capita expenditures adjusted for PPP in the health sector (Arweiler, 1997).[2]

Second, Canada's relatively high health expenditures appear to be driven more by price than by quantity. In other words, the size and use of our health infrastructure (human and physical resources) do not explain why our health expenditures are relatively high. It is the price of these resources (cost of hospital stays, remuneration of physicians and other providers) which seems to make a difference (Fournier, 1997).

Third, the way health systems are organized, financed and regulated seems to make a significant difference in cost control. At the macro level, the share of public financing in total expenditures is positively correlated with cost control. At the micro level, movement away from fee-for-service remuneration of physicians (particularly in primary care), shorter hospitalization periods and effective control over the drug costs are associated with better overall cost-control performance (Brousselle, 1997).

Finally, we found no discernible relationship between health status indicators and levels of expenditure on health care and other social programs across OECD countries, but we did find a link between health status and measures of income distribution (Sullivan, 1997). The evidence is accumulating that the higher the socio-economic status, the better the health of the individual is likely to be. Measured by income, by education or by occupation, "groups at every rung of the socio-economic ladder are healthier than those at the rung immediately below them, throughout the entire range of the socio-economic hierarchy" (Stoddart, 1995). This evidence suggests that it is not only material deprivation that causes health to deteriorate. Rather, the determinants of health are more complex, and related more to income disparities than to actual income.

Table 1: Indicators of Health Status, System Capacity and Expenditures in OECD Countries, 1994

	Life Expectancy		Premature Mortality	Demography	Hospital Inputs	Health Manpower	Total Expenditure on Health	
	Females at Birth	Males at Birth	Infant Mortality: Per 100 Live Births	Population: 65 and over	Beds: Inpatient Beds	Practising Physicians	Total Exp. on Health Share: % of GDP	Total Exp. on Health Val./Capita PPP$
	Years	Years		% Tot. Pop.	/1 000 Pop.	/1 000 Pop.		
AUSTRALIA	80.9	75.0	0.59	11.8	8.9	n/a	8.5	1606
AUSTRIA	79.7	73.3	0.63	15.0	9.4	2.6	9.7	1965
BELGIUM	79.8	73.0	0.76	15.6	7.6	3.7	8.2	1653
CANADA (rank)	81.2* (5)	74.9* (6)	0.68 (18)	11.9 (17)	6.0* (13)	2.2 (15)	9.8 (2)	2010 (3)
DENMARK	77.6	72.3	0.56	15.5	5.0	2.9	6.6	1362
FINLAND	80.2	72.8	0.46	14.2	10.1	2.7	8.3	1357
FRANCE	81.8	73.7	0.58	14.7	9.0	2.8	9.7	1866
GERMANY	79.3	73.8	0.56	15.2	9.7	3.3	9.5	1869
GREECE	79.9	74.9	0.79	14.8	5.1	4.0	5.2	598
ICELAND	80.8	77.1	0.34	11.1	n/a	3.0	8.1	1577
IRELAND	78.2*	72.7	0.59	11.5	5.0	2.0	7.9	1201
ITALY	81.2	74.7	0.66	n/a	6.7	1.7*	8.3	1561
JAPAN	83.0	76.6	0.42	14.0	15.5	1.8	6.9	1473
LUXEMBOURG	79.4	72.2	0.53	n/a	11.8	2.2	5.8	1697
MEXICO	75.8	69.4	1.70	4.1	0.8	1.3	5.3	395
NETHERLANDS	80.3	74.6	0.56	13.1	11.3	n/a	8.8	1641
NEW-ZEALAND	78.9*	73.1*	0.73	11.5	7.2*	2.1	7.5	1226
NORWAY	80.6	74.8	0.52	16.0	n/a	3.3	7.3	1604
PORTUGAL	78.2	71.2	0.81	14.4	4.3	2.9	7.6	938
SPAIN	81.0	73.3	0.60	14.8	n/a	4.1*	7.3	1005
SWEDEN	81.4	76.1	0.44	17.4	6.5	3.0	7.7	1348
SWITZERLAND	81.6	75.1	0.51	15.1	n/a	3.1	9.6	2294
UN. KINGDOM	79.5	74.2	0.62	15.7**	5.1	1.5*	6.9	1211
UNITED STATES	79.0	72.3	0.79	12.4	4.4*	2.5	14.3	3516

Source: OECD (1996). N.B. numbers in italics are 1993 data; *indicates 1992 data; **indicates 1990 data. Rankings use most recent available data for OECD countries.

Three Key Dimensions of Balance

In this section, we present a framework which sets out what we believe to be the three fundamental dimensions of balance.

Concepts and definitions are vitally important to developing a shared understanding of the challenges in resource allocation. While we did not wish to revive the age-old debate about the definition of well-being, wellness, health, and health care, we believe that a working definition of some concepts is essential to clarify our work, particularly in identifying trade-offs and establishing lines of accountability.

For ease of presentation, we have opted for a national accounts approach to illustrate the three key dimensions of balance (see Figure 1). Gross Domestic Product (GDP) represents the sum total of resources available in society to pursue health and other societal goals.[3] The sum total of these goals, "well-being", is the purview of public policy in its broadest sense and is the product of the decisions which individuals, communities and governments make every day. The health sector accounts for just under 10 percent of GDP and is primarily responsible for illness prevention and treatment. Roughly three quarters of health sector expenditures are made by governments under universal health care plans, public health programs and health research. The remainder, which includes expenditures on drugs, dental services and some components of institutional care, is privately funded, either by individuals or by business on behalf of employees.

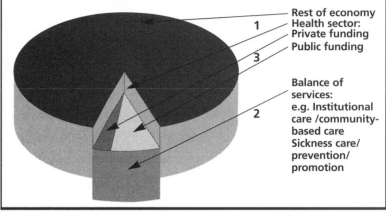

Figure 1: Dimensions of Balance

1. The health sector in relation to the rest of the economy.
2. The balance of services within the health sector.
3. The balance of funding within the health sector.

Rest of economy
Health sector:
Private funding
Public funding

Balance of services:
e.g. Institutional care /community-based care
Sickness care/ prevention/ promotion

Before going further, three observations are relevant. First, in the universe of health, there is an important distinction to be made between well-being and absence of illness. Absence of illness is not a prerequisite, nor does it automatically lead to, well-being. In our view, preventing and treating illness through effective interventions are and should continue to be the primary vocations of the health sector. Well-being, on the other hand, is a much broader concept for which no one sector of society can or should claim sole responsibility and accountability, but toward which all sectors must contribute.

Therefore, we don't think there should be a competition for resources between sickness care and promotion of well-being. Some commentators believe that pitting sickness care against health promotion, and combining the budgets for sickness care and promotion of well-being, is almost certain to favour the former. Humans have a built-in sense of their immortality, and are preoccupied by current problems rather than preventing future ones.

If society is really serious about promoting well-being and population health, there needs to be a reconfiguration of resources throughout the economy, not just the health sector. For instance, incentives should be in place to ensure that all sectors of the economy and government, in making public policy, take into consideration the health impact on persons affected by the policy change.

Second, and following from the discussion above, the boundaries between health and other sectors are not clearly delineated, particularly in the case of prevention and health promotion, as well as services for seniors, the frail elderly and the chronically ill. Both prevention and health promotion can logically be slotted either into the health sector or elsewhere depending on the nature of the programs and services falling under these general rubrics. Sophisticated social and economic interventions may well prevent certain types of morbidity even though they do not resemble, nor even have the goals of preventive health programs such as immunizations or employee fitness programs. Similarly, health promotion can take the form of what we regard as explicit health programs — anti-smoking campaigns, wellness centres—but it can also be a highly successful by-product of job creation or learning-to-read programs.

Third, GDP is based on an income/expenditure identity. That is, one dollar of expenditure on a good or service is one dollar of income for someone. Shifting the balance of expenditures therefore implies a change in the distribution of income. Reducing the relative size of the health sector means reducing incomes and/or cutting jobs in that sector, and increasing incomes and/or jobs in other sectors. The same applies for reallocations within the health sector, for example, from institutional to community-based services, or from public to privately funded services.

The equality between expenditures on health care and incomes earned from its provision is exact, following from the rules of accounting. It must be distinguished from the common observation that payments to labour — wages, salaries, and fees — make up a relatively large proportion of expenditures on health care, in contrast to, say, expenditures on food or petroleum products. The equality of income and expenditure does not, however, depend in any way on this (quite valid) observation.

The critical point is that incomes come in a number of forms, of which payment for labour (and skills) is only one. Suppose, for example, that a hospital is closed and that provincial health expenditures are reduced by the amount of its former budget. Hospital staff will lose their jobs; the connection between reduced expenditure and reduced labour income is obvious. But the other components of the budget — payments for food, drugs and other supplies — will also disappear, reducing the sales revenues of firms in those sectors. This in turn translates into reductions in their profits, and/or in the earnings of their workers and managers, and the payments to (sales revenue of) their suppliers. If profits fall, then so do the dividends (or retained earnings) of shareholders. The chain of effect may be quite long, with many branches. But at the ends of all the branches, a cut in expenditure will always result in reductions to someone's income.

Of course those who have lost sales to the hospital now closed may try to increase sales elsewhere, just as the laid-off workers may look for other jobs. But since, by hypothesis, the rest of the health care budget has not increased, this can only happen if they displace — take income away from — others in the health care sector, or if they increase sales (find jobs) outside health care. In the latter case, incomes earned from providing health care have still fallen.

Moreover, the people whose incomes are threatened by expenditure cuts, or their representatives, are very well aware of what is at stake. The long struggles in Canada over drug patents and now over provincial drug reimbursement policies have nothing to do with labour income but everything to do with drug company sales and profits. (Any alleged connection between public policy and jobs is simply part of the political bargaining.) But the drug industry defends the incomes of its shareholders — its profits — at least as fiercely as a labour union defends the incomes of its members. That is what management is paid to do.

Firms for which the health care sector represents a small share of their sales — suppliers of electricity, for example, or raw food — may not be particularly concerned about the threat from cutbacks. Their economic health has a broader base. But in general, those who are specialized sellers either of health care or to health care providers, whether they provide labour services or other commodities, will (quite correctly) see in expenditure control a significant threat to their incomes and will react accordingly.

The balance between the health sector and the rest of the economy

The literature on the determinants of health shows that the health sector is but one of many influences on the health of individuals and populations. Socioeconomic status, social supports, environmental conditions and a host of other factors have been shown to be closely associated with health status. Beyond a certain level of expenditure on health care, health status gains level off, and the opportunity cost of not investing in other determinants of health increases.

In an ideal world, policy makers would have at their disposal cost-benefit information about a broad range of public policies and could therefore pinpoint the amount of resources necessary in each sector to maximize the well-being of the population. In the real world, no such information exists. More important, even if it did, there is no consensus on how to put into operation the concept of "well-being". As a result, the relative size of the health sector and other areas of public spending is a product of a multitude of political, economic and social pressures.

Health expenditures as a share of GDP are an indicator widely used by governments and health policy analysts to track the evolution of health expenditures as a function of society's ability to pay. As we discussed earlier, it is not the only indicator of health expenditures. It is also a very cyclical indicator. For example, a recession will generally cause the ratio to increase, even if health expenditures are held well in check. Strong economic growth may lead to a decline in the ratio, even if health expenditures are on the increase. However, it is the long-term trend which is of more significance.

For the last 30 years (with the exception of the late 1970s), Canada has spent one to two percentage points more of its GDP on health compared to the average of OECD countries. Canada tracked closely with the United States until the early 1970s, at which time universal public medical insurance was adopted by all Canadian jurisdictions. Since then, US spending on health as a share of GDP has

doubled from roughly seven to 14 percent, while Canada has seen its share increase less markedly from seven to a high of about 10 percent of GDP.

However, as shown in the figure below, the most recent data from the OECD suggest that Canada has pulled back from the 10 percent threshold and is falling back in line with other industrialized countries. In 1995, Canada spent 9.5 percent of its GDP on health, well below the United States, and slightly below Austria, France and Germany.

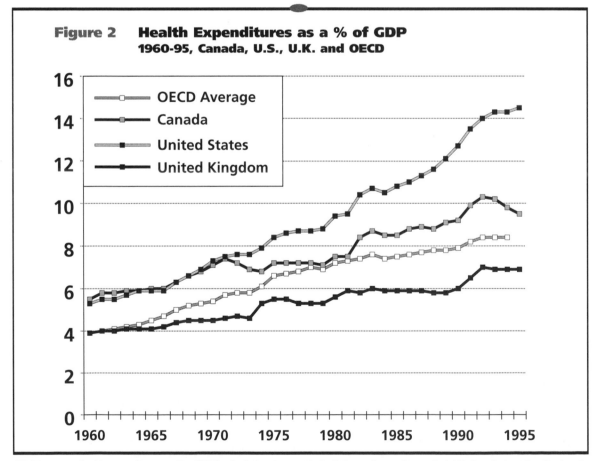

Figure 2   Health Expenditures as a % of GDP
1960-95, Canada, U.S., U.K. and OECD

OECD average health expenditures as % of GDP calculation does not include Luxembourg, Portugal and Turkey (incomplete data) and New Zealand, Mexico, Czech Republic, Hungary and Poland (staggered entry into OECD).

Against this backdrop, the two major questions in this dimension of balance are:

1) Are we spending too little or too much on our health system?

2) Are we clear on what we want the health system to achieve in an environment where the broader determinants of health merit more attention?

The balance of services within the health sector

The second dimension of balance is about the distribution of resources within the health sector. In other words, given the resources available to the health sector, what is the best configuration of services to prevent and treat illness effectively and efficiently?

Table 2 shows a breakdown of national health expenditures by category of expenditure from 1975 to 1994. During this period, total health expenditures increased by an average of 10 percent annually (approximately four percent in real terms). However, expenditures on the various categories of services did not increase evenly, resulting in changes in their relative shares. The most prominent changes are as follows:

■ There has been a shift of resources away from institutional care. This is reflected both by the significant decline in the share of health expenditures devoted to hospital services, as well as by the drop in the share of capital expenditures.

Table 2: Breakdown of National Health Expenditures by Category of Expenditure, 1975-1994.

	1975		1994	
	$million	%	$million	%
Hospitals	5,512	44.9	26,999	37.2
Other institutions	1,124	9.2	7,090	9.8
Physicians	1,840	15.0	10,323	14.2
Other professionals	902	7.3	6,193	8.5
Drugs	1,074	8.8	9,179	12.7
Public health	515	4.2	3,618	5.0
Home care	320	0.3	1,024	1.4
Capital	537	4.4	2,074	2.9
Other	720	5.9	5,962	8.2
Total	**12,265**	**100.0**	**72,463**	**100.0**

Source: National Health Expenditures in Canada, 1975-94. Numbers may not add up due to rounding.

- Drugs have increased their share dramatically from about nine to 13 percent of health expenditures. While this includes prescription and non-prescription drugs, as well as other personal health products, the trend is what is important.

- Some areas of expenditure have increased their share only marginally. These include other institutions (mostly nursing homes for seniors), other professionals (dentists, chiropractors, physiotherapists, etc.), home care, public health and "other expenditures" (a catch-all category).

What lies behind these changes? Have we gone too far in some cases, not far enough in others? Later in this report, we shall examine a number of these shifts in more detail (pharmaceutical issues, as mentioned earlier, are explored in a separate report). We have also devoted some attention to the organizational features of our health system insofar as they influence the balance of services within the system.

. . . private health care financing can distort resource allocation by creating excess capacity, and by skewing resources toward high-tech services and administrative machinery.

The public/private balance within the health sector

The third dimension of balance is primarily about how services delivered by the health sector are financed. This has important ramifications for both dimensions of balance discussed above. As we shall discuss further, and as our commissioned work has clearly shown (see Deber et al., 1997), at the broader societal level, an over-reliance on private health care financing tends to unnecessarily inflate health expenditures, thereby crowding out other worthwhile expenditures in other sectors. Within the health sector, private health care financing can distort resource allocation by creating excess capacity, and by skewing resources toward high-tech services and administrative machinery.

Over the last two decades, the share of private financing has increased gradually from 25 percent to 28 percent of total health expenditures. This has led many experts, analysts and observers to conclude that our health care system is slowly being privatized. A number of commentators have even concluded that we no longer have a single-tier system whereby everybody is provided services based on need rather than ability to pay.

Table 3 provides a breakdown of health expenditures by source of financing: "public" mainly comprises general tax revenues, whereas "private" includes premiums for private insurance, co-payments, deductibles and out-of-pocket expenditures. The data present an interesting story often buried underneath the aggregate numbers.

Table 3: Breakdown of Health Expenditures by Financial Source, 1975 - 1994

	1975			1994			Avg. Annual Compounded Growth, '75-'94	
	Public $million	Private $million	Ratio $million	Public $million	Private $million	Ratio	Public (%)	Priv. (%)
Hospitals	5,196	316	94:6	24,206	2,793	90:10	8.4	12.2
Other inst.	796	328	71:29	4,952	2,138	70:30	10.1	10.4
Physicians	1,813	27	99:1	10,222	100	99:1	9.5	7.1
Other prof'ls	135	766	15:85	847	5,346	14:86	10.1	10.8
Drugs	158	916	15:85	2,929	6,250	32:68	16.6	10.6
Other	1,264	540	70:30	8,905	3,773	70:30	10.8	10.8
Total	9,361	2,893	76:24	52,061	20,401	72:28	9.5	10.8

Source: National Health Expenditures in Canada, 1975-94. Numbers may not add up due to rounding.

First, public financing in our system is concentrated on hospital and physician services. Together, these two areas account for over 55 percent of public funding. This "single-tier" system guarantees equal access to Canadians, based on need. In addition, there are large public outlays in areas beyond the mandate of the *Canada Health Act*.

Second, while overall, private expenditures have been growing marginally faster than public expenditures, this is not the case for all areas of expenditure. In particular, public outlays for drugs have been growing at a much faster rate than private expenditures. This can be traced to the expansion of provincial drug insurance plans during the late 1970s and early 1980s.

Finally, in only one area — hospitals — has growth in private spending from 1975 to 1994 significantly outstripped growth in public spending. Private financing in this area is limited to upgraded accommodation, revenues from parking, cafeterias and concessions, investment income, private fund raising, services to non-insured persons and procedures which are not deemed medically necessary[4]—hardly what one would equate with privatization of our health care system.

That is not to say that all is well in the private/public balance. For medically necessary hospital and physician services, the current regime has worked fairly well. There are no user charges, private insurance is implicitly or explicitly forbidden and there is no opting-out of paying taxes for the public system. However, there is a perception among providers and the public that access to core services is deteriorating, and that access to needed drug therapies, home care and other emerging types of services is wanting. There is the question of private versus public delivery of services (some would call this contracting out of publicly funded services) which tends to seep into the debate about public and private financing from time to time. Then there is the issue of whether to define "medical necessity" more clearly to distinguish core services from other services.

We believe that in principle all medically necessary services should be publicly funded. In practice this is hard to achieve, but still should be the strategic direction guiding decisions. At a First Minister's conference in Ottawa in 1965 convened to discuss health services, Lester B. Pearson, in a speech to delegates, offered support for extensive public coverage. "The scope of benefits should be, broadly speaking, all the services provided by physicians, both general practitioners and specialists. A complete health plan would include dental treatment, prescribed drugs, and other important services, and there is nothing in the approach we propose to prevent these being included, from the start or later, if this were the general wish. We regard comprehensive physicians' services as the initial minimum" (Pearson, 1965). As we shall argue in the final section of this report, we need to take appropriate steps to reinforce the role of public financing in our health care system.

Rebalancing at the Societal Level

A clearer mission for Canada's health system

If achieving the best health possible for the population as a whole with minimal or no disparities were the dominant public policy objective, our society might be organized in a much different fashion than it is today. Our tax system would be much more progressive, income disparities would be significantly reduced, policies in all areas would be geared toward prevention and risk reduction, children and families would be more highly valued, and poverty and unemployment would truly become Public Enemies Number One and Two. Whether we would be individually or collectively more or less wealthy than we are today is not entirely clear, but the literature on the determinants of health suggests that we would probably be healthier. But would we still need to have a high-quality system of universal health care? We believe so.

There is a very old debate in philosophy about "utilitarianism" which is central to the issue of balance. The debate hinges on the following question: Under what circumstances is it justified to overlook individual needs and rights to maximize "utility" at the societal level? In the area of health, the question might be more aptly posed as: Under what circumstances is it justified to deny effective health care to an individual in need to improve the health prospects of others in society? Fortunately, it is a question of distributive justice with which we are not often explicitly confronted.[5] However, the population health perspective does shift our thinking in the direction of

utilitarianism precisely because it draws attention to the opportunity costs of health care expenditures — spending thousands of dollars on open heart surgery might improve the health prospects of an individual, while spending the same amount on early childhood education may significantly improve the health prospects of one or more individuals.

The analogy with the criminal justice system is powerful. As a society, we have decided that any individual accused of having committed a crime has a right to a fair trial. It does not matter that trials and incarceration are expensive, nor that resources might be more effectively deployed to prevent crime from happening in the first place. The right to a fair trial is a fundamental principle of justice in our society. Similarly, our health care system has been built around the notion, which we strongly support, that no one should be denied effective health care when in need.

That being said, prevention of adverse outcomes in the areas of health and crime is a worthwhile pursuit. Given that the concept of "need" is more difficult to define in such circumstances, we would suggest that investment of public monies at this level be guided by the ability-to-benefit principle. However, what is emerging from the growing body of knowledge on determinants of health is that doing something to prevent adverse health outcomes equates with doing something to prevent adverse life outcomes, which no one sector has the mandate or the resources to accomplish.

Good, socially responsible public policy in a broad range of areas is conducive to better health outcomes. In the health sector, we might call this healthy public policy. It is also likely to be conducive to better outcomes in the areas of crime prevention, education and social integration. But regardless of what can be accomplished by acting on the determinants of adverse life outcomes, people will still need access to health care, a fair trial, a basic education and a social safety net.

As we turn our attention toward improving population health, we must be clear about what we wish to accomplish, and we must never sacrifice the very system Canadians have grown to cherish. The health sector can play a very effective role as an advocate for, and partner in, strategies which act on the basic determinants of health. But we must resist the temptation of taking on too broad of a mandate for achieving health objectives.

The bottom line is that distributing money and power is the same as distributing health status. We should not hold health authorities accountable for reducing inequities in health. But we should hold them accountable for identifying needs, clarifying connections, and telling the truth about why some people are healthy and others are not.

The bottom line is that distributing money and power is the same as distributing health status. We should not hold health authorities accountable for reducing inequities in health. But we should hold them accountable for identifying needs, clarifying connections, and telling the truth about why some people are healthy and others are not.

Moreover, we believe that there is a shared agenda for implementing a broad range of public policy interventions which could improve population health. One of the most important messages emerging from the work of the Determinants of Health Working Group is the need to find effective ways of fostering intersectoral collaboration. At the local level, there are many examples of successful inter-sectoral collaboration. At higher levels of government, the challenge becomes greater and more complicated, and successful examples are fewer. However, if we do want to develop a capacity to replicate some of the Determinants of Health Working Group's success stories on a larger scale, it will be critical to establish mechanisms at all levels of government to support multisectoral policy development and programming. In the early 1980s, the now defunct Ministry of State for Social Development had such a mandate at the national level. Ontario's Premier's Council on Health, Well-Being and Social Justice was a similar mechanism at the provincial level, though it did not oversee any spending. Some jurisdictions have also adopted a mandatory health impact assessment in the development of all public policies.

Perhaps the best we can do at this stage is to continue experimenting with different ways of fostering intersectoral collaboration, while ensuring that an appropriate infrastructure is in place to produce, disseminate and analyze the growing body of information on population health. Resources are too scarce and problems are becoming too complex to keep our old ways.

The Working Group on Striking a Balance therefore recommends:

a) *That the Conference of Federal/ Provincial/Territorial Ministers of Health articulate a national health policy framework for the 21st century which clearly establishes that the primary mission of the health sector is first to prevent and treat illness according to the fundamental principles of medicare, and second to collaborate with other sectors in the development of population health interventions which have the most potential to improve the health of Canadians.*

b) *That all jurisdictions promote a population health agenda by:*

— *supporting the nation-wide health information system proposed by the Evidence-Based Decision Making Working Group; and*

— *taking steps within governments, to develop appropriate budgetary, decision-making and policy development structures to facilitate intersectoral collaboration that will ultimately link a broad range of economic and social portfolios as a means of promoting a population health agenda.*

Are we spending too much or too little on health care?

There is a constant debate in the Canadian health care system on whether it has enough money. This is hardly surprising, since there are tens of thousands of board members, managers and practitioners who are preoccupied with this question at regular intervals as they carry out their tasks. Furthermore, because the system is largely public, politicians and citizens turn their attention to this question on a formal basis as part of the electoral process.

The question grows in importance when the funding environment shifts gears. Beginning in the late 1980s, and accelerating in the 1990s, governments have challenged the notion that the health sector budget should perpetually grow in real terms. In absolute terms, the health sector has not been particularly hard hit. Only during the last two years has the percentage of GDP devoted to health spending declined. Other industries, such as farming on the prairies and the steel industry, have suffered massive job losses and undergone often traumatic restructuring in the last 10 to 20 years. But the world is made up of relative perceptions as well as absolutes; in relative terms, the 1990s have been quite tough on the health sector, particularly that part funded through the tax system. The question, then, is unusually interesting at this time. Before we offer our answer, it is worthwhile to review the environment in which the question is posed, and the elements of a cogent answer.

First, the health system does not have enough money if one expects a perpetual growth in the number of people working in the system and the number and range of services delivered. A system that is frozen at a certain level or even somewhat reduced will not fulfil this expectation unless the unit price of services drops to allow for greater volumes and range. In the health sector, most costs are labour, and history tells us labour costs do not generally drop. While some technology costs do get lower — such as CT scanners — there are always new and more expensive technologies clamouring for a place, pushing up costs. It is inevitable that when new constraints are introduced, someone will be unhappy, particularly the provider or the consumer who will feel the effects of the changes most directly. If we measure the system by the amount of happiness observed in providers and consumers, we will invariably conclude that the quality of the system has declined when constraints are imposed. But the system does not exist to maximize the happiness of those who provide services and those who receive them. It exists to meet real needs, and an implicit goal is to meet these needs at the least possible cost so that other needs and desires can be fulfilled as well.

. . . the system does not exist to maximize the happiness of those who provide services and those who receive them. It exists to meet real needs . . .

Second, everyone who works in a particular sector has a natural interest in its expansion, both in absolute and relative terms. More than a million Canadians earn their living from the health care system. Their desire to expand its scope, technological capabilities and impact is both understandable and admirable. Likewise, it is only to be expected that they will vociferously oppose cutbacks, both because they may genuinely think that public health will be adversely affected, and certainly because these cuts constitute a threat to the livelihood of many of their colleagues, and often themselves. These same providers are the main sources of information and education for the public. Most citizens are not in a position to make fully informed decisions about how much health care the population needs, and they tend to pay attention to providers arguing the general case just as they pay attention to providers in day-to-day health encounters. Just like every other sector, the health sector and its workers will pursue their own interests and claim these to be identical with the public interest in all cases. But society has long recognized that particular and general interests do not always coincide, and it is important to examine thoroughly to what extent the claims and desires of the health care sector are about its own self-interest rather than the public's.

Third, it has always been extremely difficult to identify causal links between expenditure levels, cutbacks and adverse health events, particularly in a large and historically well-funded health system. It is true that bad things happen to sick people, and it is also true that some people are badly served in the health care system. When these things coincide with the imposition of financial restraint, many will argue that the restraint caused the adverse event. But adverse events took place when the system was growing rapidly. We also know that there is a considerable amount of inefficiency in the health system in the form of unnecessary procedures, inappropriate use of

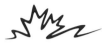

resources and ineffective treatment. Resources can be managed well or managed poorly.

Fourth, there is a great deal of rhetoric about the reputed decline in system quality. In fact we do not have any valid and comprehensive measure of the quality of the health care system. Certainly a well-run system with a lot of money can provide a better-quality service than a well-run system with a lot less money. But there is considerable evidence showing that variations in practice account for a far greater proportion of observable quality problems than the absolute amount of money in the system. The literature on quality assurance, total quality management and continuous quality improvement makes very few references to the absolute amount of money in a system. These practice variations not only result in poor or inappropriate service for many people, but they also tend to push up costs because in most cases, poor service is also inefficient service.

Fifth, poor quality can be the result of both not enough service and too much service. Accessibility is in itself no confirmation of quality; indeed, some services are demonstrably too accessible, with adverse health results. For instance, overprescribing of antibiotics has led to the emergence of resistant strains of bacteria that render the drugs less effective. Too many nursing homes may lead to unnecessary admissions and loss of autonomy and capacity among elderly people who could have stayed in the community. Unconstrained access to Caesarean section and lack of encouragement for vaginal births in subsequent pregnancies may result in unnecessary surgery as well as

higher costs. Overscreening for the presence of prostate cancer may result in investigation and interventions for many men who never would have died from the disease but who may suffer extremely high complication rates associated with interventions such as surgery.

Sixth, an unhappy system probably does result in diminished quality, and certainly conveys the impression to the public that things are going downhill. Low morale does not necessarily mean that a system does not have enough money. But it may be a sign of a system that has not successfully communicated to its workers and the public the need for, and advantages of, change. Furthermore, large and complex human systems can sustain only a certain pace of change without showing serious strains.

More fundamentally, the question of "how much money should we spend" is logically related to the question of "what do we want to achieve". What we want to achieve is multidimensional . . .

Given these factors, the question of whether or not there is enough money in the Canadian health system is unanswerable. By world standards, our system has been richly funded throughout the last several decades. We have always spent as much or more money than the average of the most advanced nations in the world, and until recently held down second place to the United States. Our unit costs have been relatively high, no doubt influenced by forces south of the border. More fundamentally, the question of "how much money should we spend" is logically related to the question of "what do we want to achieve". What we want to achieve is multidimensional: fairness, efficiency, effective interventions, creativity, high service standards, well-trained personnel, and a discerning public. While there are several good measures of individual service quality related to satisfaction, process and outcome, we do not have total system indicators. On a 100-point scale, we do not know whether our system rates a 50, an 80 or a 96. There are polling figures suggesting that the public perceives that the quality of the system has declined recently, but there are no objective measures verifying this, and these responses are hardly surprising given the messages of doom and gloom emanating from the critics of restraint.

Having said this, it is quite possible that the system is not as good as it once was. Managing people and deploying resources are doubtless more difficult under conditions of restraint than continuous growth. If the system operates pretty much in the same old way, but in a far more strained fiscal environment, there is no guarantee that the ineffective services will be the first to go. In the absence of information allowing good decisions to be made about which services should remain and be enhanced, and which are nonessential, there will be a tendency for across-the-board cuts that eliminate the good and the useful as well as the useless.

Canadians are concerned about the pace at which funds are being withdrawn from the system — and the consequent downsizing. The variation in service availability across provinces and territories has alerted the public

to the impact of federal cuts, but there are few objective measures available. Governments should develop indicators to permit monitoring of the changes in the system and their impact on health outcomes. With these indicators as guides, provinces can work with the federal government, providers and the public to determine both the direction and pace of change.

It is important to note that the performance of the overall system can only be as good as the people working in it. If there is widespread discontent, ongoing fears about job security, real or perceived arbitrariness in the way cuts are made and the pace at which they are achieved, and conflict among government, managers and providers, the discontent will show up in some diminished service quality. It is perhaps noteworthy that the two provinces that appear to be experiencing the greatest levels of public and provider discontent are precisely those whose expenditure levels have been among the highest in recent years — Ontario and Alberta.[6] Managing the change and building a sense of commitment to a new way of doing business are prerequisites to successful health reform, especially in that restraint is always a disheartening element of restructuring.

Similarly, disagreements about the amount of money in the system are often disagreements about fundamental values. Those who opt for restraint maintain that the health care system is a service industry that in itself has limited capacity to create wealth, while those who favour its growth argue that it is an investment in human capital that pays huge returns. Those who want continual expansion believe that health care services are the hallmark of a successful and prosperous society, and greater consumption is intrinsically good. Others argue that self-reliance and maintaining control of one's own health are dangerously neglected virtues, and that an over-abundance of health care services unintentionally creates dependencies.

The Working Group on Striking a Balance has identified the following functions as important in order to improve accountability and transparency of the health care system:

a) Collection of timely information to track and process the impact of health care reforms and reductions in health care funding.

b) Development of quality of care, health outcome, and patient satisfaction outcome indicators comparable across provinces and territories, and regions.

c) Distribution of the information in a) and b) to governments, government authorities and the public, in a systematic way.

Rebalancing Within the Health Sector

Shifting toward non-institutional care

The balance within the health care sector has in recent years shifted toward non-institutional care. This has taken three main forms:

- an increase in home care and other community-based services, and a reduction in the use of inpatient hospital services in favour of day or outpatient services;

- the reduction or elimination of particularly lighter-care nursing home beds in favour of home care and congregate housing;

- an emphasis on "wellness" services such as prevention and health promotion.

These shifts have distinct characteristics, and we address them separately below.

a) Acute care substitution

There has been a gradual decline in inpatient hospitalization rates over the last 10 years. Many inpatient surgical procedures are now done on a day basis, examples being cataract removal and lens replacement, and arthroscopic joint surgery. Pre-admission outpatient clinics have replaced the one- to three-day inpatient stays prior to surgery. New mothers and their babies typically return home in one to three days instead of spending five to seven days in hospital. Convalescent periods in hospital are constantly being reduced through discharge planning programs and the expansion of home care. Two province-wide studies (in Saskatchewan and Manitoba) have shown that a large proportion of hospital days continue to be used by people who do not require acute care. (Health Services Utilization and Research Commission, 1994; DeCoster C. et al., 1996).

While many have expressed concerns about the nature and extent of these shifts, there is no evidence that reduced stays in hospitals have adversely affected health status or readmission rates. Initial results from Manitoba showed that hospitals with the lowest length of stay for various diagnoses also had the lowest rates of readmission. There are anecdotal concerns raised by patients and providers that home care is insufficiently developed to provide safe and comprehensive service to people discharged early from hospital. Statements about newborn re-admissions can and should be documented and evaluated, and comparisons made with geographical areas with lower re-admission rates. However, these concerns may result from the transformation of hospitals to facilities used when all other options have been exhausted instead of the primary site of both intense services and convalescence. Without question, patients and their families express a preference for day surgery and minimally invasive surgery that reduce or eliminate inpatient stays, allowing a return to either the home or the work force (or both).

While the number of patient days per thousand population is substantially below 1,000 annually in most jurisdictions, Canada's rates remain higher than in many areas of the United States. It is notable that target rates established by royal commissions or their

equivalents tend to be surpassed sooner than expected. It is, of course, possible to discharge prematurely, with adverse consequences. Very likely there are cases where people have been sent home too soon, but this has always been the case in an imperfect system. It should be possible to monitor the consequences of reduced hospital stays using administrative and other evaluative data. In addition, it should be possible to develop indicators on whether the hospital system has off-loaded responsibility prematurely.

Finally, acute care substitution is essentially an efficiency concept: the assumption is that outcomes and satisfaction levels will be the same (or better), but costs will be lower. Both costs and outcomes should be quite measurable. If there is lingering debate about the appropriateness of reducing the emphasis on hospital care, they are resolvable empirically. It is not only a question of whether services are required, but whether they are most effectively and efficiently delivered. However, regardless of how quickly new technology is changing the role of hospitals, there is always a lag in actual adjustments to human and physical resources.

b) Long-term care substitution

Although international comparisons are notoriously difficult because of non-standardized definitions of long-term care beds, historically Canada has been a high user. Where other countries have opted for expanded home care and/or housing units with built-in features to accommodate elderly people, the Canadian response has been to build long-term care facilities. In a fragmented system with a major private component, long-term care facilities maintain their own waiting lists and apply their own admissions criteria. Regionalization and the development of mandatory, co-ordinated assessment and placement protocols have reduced or eliminated waiting lists, ensured that those in greatest need have priority access to vacant beds, and in general lowered the institutionalization rate considerably (New Brunswick, 1991; Alberta Health, 1994).

The expansion of home care, particularly where it is fully integrated with the other parts of the health system, has substantially reduced the need for admission to long-term care facilities. One concern is whether the lower institutionalization rates have been achieved by shifting the burden of care from the public system to individuals and their families. The issue here is both financial and philosophical: it is relatively straightforward to calculate whether or not it costs more to keep someone at home than in an institution, but it becomes more complex to determine whether it is the right thing to do when one factors in the financial and non-financial impact on the family caregivers and other non-monetary considerations. Nonetheless, the direction is appropriate given Canada's traditionally high utilization rates. Again, we do not yet have indicators to signal when community care and families are becoming overwhelmed, although good assessment tools do take full account of the home environment and the capabilities and propensities of caregivers.

c) Health promotion, public health, and wellness

There is a good deal of confusion surrounding the concept of a "wellness," as opposed to a "sickness," model of health services, and the distinction between health promotion and prevention. These concepts and uncertainties are not new. Both Lalonde (1974) and Epp (1986) advocated a "positive health" perspective to complement sickness care. All provincial royal commissions came to essentially the same conclusion. There is a long and strong intellectual tradition in Canada that encompasses the desirability of health maintenance and enhancement through non-medical interventions, and a recognition that the health of the population is linked to a much broader set of determinants than health care. Nonetheless, there are widespread concerns about the role of health promotion and prevention programs in the overall context of health services, and the criteria used to assess whether this wellness shift is likely to be effective.

We have two principal conclusions on these subjects. First, evaluation and accountability criteria must be appropriate to the programs and services in question. This means that, for example, health promotion programs ought to be subject to the same rigorous scrutiny as sickness care programs. The goals of these programs must be articulated, and the complexity of the relationship between expenditures, services and outcomes, must be acknowledged. Furthermore, we must recognize that prevention and health promotion programs do not affect all segments of the population equally. In particular, disadvantaged groups are often the main potential beneficiaries of health promotion and prevention activities, but for various reasons it may be difficult to reach the target groups effectively given the strength of such forces as lack of education, low income and high unemployment rates. There may also be a significant time lag between the intervention and the final outcome, mediated by many confounding factors. To some this suggests that we should pursue health promotion programs as an act of faith. Our view is that we should vigorously develop sophisticated evaluation and accountability indicators so that eventually, we can target services more effectively and establish a solid empirical basis for increasing funding and emphasis.

Second, positing a competition between health and health care does not serve us well. Sickness care is the cornerstone of what we think of as medicare. Our consultations revealed a profound understanding among the public of the determinants of health and the limits to health care. Yet people fear the erosion of the sickness care system, and do not wish to be forced into a situation where they must choose between promotion and prevention on the one hand, and sickness care on the other. We cannot say what the balance in expenditures should be between health promotion, prevention and sickness care, but we do know that without assurance that needed sickness care will be available when

. . . without assurance that needed sickness care will be available when required, there will be little enthusiasm for even the most effective health promotion and prevention interventions.

required, there will be little enthusiasm for even the most effective health promotion and prevention interventions.

The Working Group on Striking a Balance therefore recommends:

a) That administrative data and standardized evaluation methods be developed to indicate whether the hospital system has off-loaded responsibility, and to signal an unsustainable shift to community care and families.

b) As part of the health research agenda recommended by the Evidence-Based Decision Making group, that rigorous evaluation of health promotion, disease prevention, and sickness care interventions be pursued using methods appropriate to the topics of inquiry.

Health system organization — in search of the magic bullet

In this section, we review three distinct, but closely related organizational features of health systems: decentralization, integration and allocation mechanisms. Our underlying assumption, borne out by the sheer number of experiments occurring at home and abroad, is that these features may hold the most potential to achieve a successful rebalancing within the health sector.

Various combinations and permutations of these features can be found in jurisdictions across Canada and abroad. However, it is not our intent to review or advise on any particular model of health system organization. Rather, we hope to contribute to ongoing discussions by flagging what we believe are the merits and trade-offs associated with further change in each of the following three areas.

a) Decentralization

For a variety of historical, constitutional and practical reasons, health care delivery is already very decentralized in Canada. Since provinces have constitutional responsibility for the organization and delivery of health services, they are responsible for roughly two thirds of public health expenditures (or about half of total health expenditures). The federal government's role is primarily centred on the regulation of drugs and devices, provision of health services to certain groups (Indians on reserves, RCMP and the Canadian Armed Forces), research funding, disease surveillance, health promotion and prevention, and maintenance of national health care principles under the mandate of the *Canada Health Act*. Cash and tax transfers to provinces in 1994 under Established Programs Financing amounted to approximately 30 percent of publicly funded health expenditures, or 22 percent of total health expenditures. About half was in the form of cash. The recently introduced Canada Health and Social Transfer (CHST) merged federal funding for health, post-secondary education and welfare into one lump sum, with a minimum cash floor of $11.1 billion. Federal direct expenditures on health (excluding transfers to provinces) amount to approximately five percent of public health expenditures (or about 3.5 percent of total expenditures).

Over the last five years or so, several provinces have taken initiatives to further decentralize the management of their respective systems through regionalization initiatives. Although not all identical, each initiative involves some degree of decentralization of decision making at the sub-provincial level. It is a move which is intended to give local authorities and communities a greater say in how health funding is allocated.

In summary, our health care system is characterized by *political decentralization* at the national level, and by *administrative decentralization* at the provincial level (Contandriopoulos, A.P. et al., 1996). Political decentralization provides provincial governments with the latitude they need to fund and manage their health care systems effectively in accordance with the broad principles of the *Canada Health Act*. Administrative decentralization at the provincial level allows provincial governments to control financing, while giving a greater say to local authorities about how resources should be allocated.

Is there a need for further decentralization at the national or provincial levels? Participants in the Forum's consultation process strongly endorsed the need to preserve national health care principles and a continuation of transfer payments to provinces. At the same time, a slight majority of participants supported a move toward greater regionalization and decentralization in the form of regional health authorities and community or district health councils, albeit with caveats and cautions.

> *"Indeed, virtually every analysis that argues that a federal role exists also argues that money is the only effective lever. ... Even in other federated countries, which accord greater regulatory powers in health to the central government than does Canada, financial participation is generally the most or one of the most important instruments of the national government." (Maslove, 1996)*

We agree with at least part of this assessment. At the national level, more decentralization really means abandoning the principles of the *Canada Health Act,* or otherwise relying on the collective will of the provinces to develop and maintain a set of national principles. There is no viable alternative to federal-provincial transfers if we are truly serious about maintaining national health care principles as we know them. Interprovincial agreements, despite best intentions, would likely evolve toward an increasingly minimalist interpretation of national requirements as provinces, over time, experience different economic circumstances, priorities and political preferences. As well, health and finance policy-makers should take note of public concerns that the cash transfer level may be less effective than it once was with respect to maintaining national standards.

Further decentralization at the provincial level would imply moving toward a form of political decentralization. Regions might be able to raise funds, and locally elected representatives would be formally responsible for resource allocation decisions. As we shall elaborate further, there is a great deal more that can be done to improve resource allocation through integration and allocation mechanisms without creating another level of government and an additional layer of bureaucracy.

Our conclusion in this area is as follows:

- First, maintaining broad national principles for health care is not incompatible with a decentralized health care delivery system. Decentralization should not be viewed as an "all or nothing" issue. There is no paradox in maintaining a federal role in a decentralized system. We say yes to reducing overlap and duplication, but we also support shared federal-provincial responsibility.

- Second, with shared responsibility should flow shared commitment and accountability. Some argue that the reduction in federal contributions to health signals federal disengagement from health. While we welcome the federal government's announcement in 1996 to establish a cash floor for CHST transfers to provinces, the federal government's need to get its fiscal house in order must be balanced against the need for provinces to have an adequate and stable resource base to fund health services. We do not doubt that additional efficiencies can be achieved in the health sector over time, however, there is a limit to how quickly the system can absorb cuts, whether they originate at the federal or provincial level. To our knowledge, decisions about future levels of federal-provincial transfers have not been based on such considerations. Unilateral federal cuts should not drive the pace or direction of change in provincial systems.

■ Third, administrative decentralization at the provincial level carries both opportunities and risks for rebalancing. Providing that provinces retain the authority and accountability for defining eligibility, coverage and benefits, there is potential for a better match between resources and regional and local needs. However, if the infrastructure and expertise are not present at the regional level, the resource allocation process may be overtaken by interest groups. This underlines the importance of thoroughly evaluating the experience of all jurisdictions in this regard.

b) Integration

Despite initiatives to restructure and regionalize health services in most provinces, the health system continues to a large extent to be organized on a "silo" basis, with a few notable pockets of integration. Of course, there will always be silos. The challenge is to build coordinating mechanisms and incentives to offset their impact. One province, Prince Edward Island, has established regions with an integrated budgetary and decision-making structure for health care institutions, community health services, social services, some justice services and housing. Health and social services are, to a certain extent, integrated in Quebec and New Brunswick. However, in all cases, funding and decision-making structures for physician services and drug programs have largely remained centralized at the provincial

level. Other services which are typically not well integrated within the system (albeit with significant variation across the country) include specialized diagnostic and institutional services, mental health and psychiatric services, public health and home care.

During public consultations, the Working Group heard an outpouring of concern about community care, home care services and pharmaceutical coverage. As a result of the increasing proportion of elderly persons in Canada, increasing numbers of two-income households, as well as greater awareness of the needs of the elderly, many members of the public think of long-term care and home care provision as being equally essential as doctors and hospitals, and as vital components of care.

Unilateral federal cuts should not drive the pace or direction of change in provincial systems.

Hospital administrators and policy makers prefer hospitals to serve the purpose for which they were designed: to treat patients with acute conditions in need of acute and intensive care and supervision. Hospitals are monitoring patients more carefully to determine when it would be suitable to treat them in less costly environments. However, medicare — because it covers in-hospital care (including medical services and supplies) — becomes an incentive to keep patients in hospital, rather than to find alternative care settings.

Decision makers in the federal-provincial arena are discussing primary care reform as a means of changing the incentive system within which physicians and other primary care providers function[7]. Primary care reform is intended to integrate components of care that at present are too compartmentalized. In some cases, such as continuing care, this will involve linking various sites for recuperative care, or strengthening current links. Integration does not necessarily mean that one organization owns and manages the various components of the system, but that it has responsibility (funding and accountability) to purchase or provide services for a defined population.

Participants in the Forum's public consultations arrived at a high degree of consensus on the characteristics of an integrated system. It should be community-based, offer an array of services, and be staffed by multidisciplinary providers. Most participants thought that a variety of personnel and system components such as nurses, physicians, other providers, health institutions and social service agencies should be linked.

If there are going to be "single points of access" to teams of providers and services, financial incentives will have to be in place to encourage significant reorganization of our current system. One means of linking the delivery of health services is to integrate funding streams through population-based funding approaches[8] and to give regions responsibility for providing a broad range of services to their population. A second entails the creation of autonomous but publicly accountable organizations which would receive population-based funding to provide a full range of health services to its members (i.e. enrolment would be voluntary or geographically driven, or a combination of both).

Movement toward integrated structures at the regional level is a key feature of most provincial organizational reform initiatives. For example, Saskatchewan's district health boards are now responsible for funding and/or providing community health services, home care, long-term care, mental and public health services and hospital care. What is missing in all cases, at this stage of evolution, is physician services (except those in community health centres), and in some cases, tertiary hospital and other specialized services.

"Introducing and supporting models with a greater service orientation and a more intimate relationship to the population they serve, with strong incentives for responsiveness and advocacy on their behalf, provide a powerful demonstration of government's fulfilment of its commitment to the people."
(Marriott and Mable, 1997)

Although Canada has had little experience with the second approach, a strong case can be made for the development of integrated organizations which would receive capitated funding to provide a full range of health services to a rostered population, along the lines of the Comprehensive Health Organization now being piloted in a couple of Ontario communities (Marriott and Mable, 1997). In a way, these models are not dissimilar to regional authorities funded on an adjusted per capita base. However, they are not geographically driven; in urban areas, they could "compete" against each other. Furthermore, they would be more independent from government

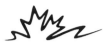

(but still very much accountable to government) and would have considerable scope to negotiate contracts with providers. While the model could be used within or as an alternative to regionalized models, there may be other applications, for example for specialized disease groups such as HIV/AIDS patients, the frail elderly, children, or for Aboriginal communities wishing to develop their own health system.[9]

Of course, no restructuring would be complete without revisiting the scope of practice of providers. We are already seeing more community based services. Advances in health technology and pharmaceutical development will catalyze movement of patients from institutional to other care settings. Consequently, planning for human resources in Canada must be consistent with these changes. The barriers, however, are formidable. Health sector employees have entrenched interests in relation to the duties they perform, the level of responsibility they undertake, and the job itself. Any of these is vulnerable during a process of reengineering, and therefore, the professional colleges, unions and associations are thrust into competition with each other. Administratively, if new categories of health professionals do emerge, professional standards, competency guidelines, licensing requirements, and training/education programs must be developed.

It has been suggested (Pew Health Professions Commission, 1995) that reform in this country will follow the movement of reform in the United States, including re-engineering of the hospital workforce, and an increase in demand for public health professionals and epidemiologists. Certainly the way we educate medical professionals will require fundamental changes with respect to research and patient care.

Industrial restructuring invariably involves looking at the distribution of work, and so too should the health sector be subjected to a thorough and rational review. The bottom line is that the success of health system renewal efforts will depend to a large extent on the 'fit' between health human resource policy and new delivery models.

The bottom line is that the success of health system renewal efforts will depend to a large extent on the 'fit' between health human resource policy and new delivery models

c) Allocation mechanisms

Allocation mechanisms refer to the basis upon which funding is distributed to health service providers. In publicly financed health care systems, there are two basic options:

1) *Patient follows money:*
   Government planners decide where particular services will be provided and fund such services based on agreed upon rules (e.g., global budgets for hospitals). Patients must go wherever the services happen to be.

2) *Money follows patient:* Funding is allocated to providers based on their ability to attract clients (e.g., fee-for-service payment for physician services).

Although payment mechanisms have received a great deal of attention in Canada over the years, the way providers in the health care system are remunerated has not changed significantly: hospitals are largely funded via prospective global budgets; physicians are still mostly paid by fee-for-service with collective and/or individual caps; and pharmacists are paid on a fee-for-service basis (except hospital pharmacists, who are on salary).

In recent months, as discussed in the preceding section, there has been renewed interest in reforming the structure and funding of primary care in Canada, and there is an ongoing interest in performance-based hospital funding. Recent reforms in New Zealand and some European countries (for example, the United Kingdom and the Netherlands) have tried to foster more competitive behaviour by having public authorities tender contracts for a full range of health services. In health policy jargon, this is called "internal markets". Others (for example, Sweden) have opted to give citizens a greater say in where health dollars are spent by instituting a system whereby patients are free to choose their providers. Health policy jargon for this approach is "public competition". So far, jurisdictions across the country have resisted the temptation to adopt competitive mechanisms such as these.

Other than some discussion of the pros and cons of fee-for-service for physicians, the Forum's public consultations did not broach in any depth different modes of funding providers. There is, however, a broad recognition of the need to make the necessary changes to put patients, rather than providers, at the centre of the system. Consultations with stakeholders did provide an opportunity to discuss funding mechanisms, including market-driven approaches. On the issue of

planned market models as practiced in some European countries, stakeholders agreed that a thorough evaluation must take place before considering their adoption in the Canadian context. Concerns were raised about the applicability of internal market approaches in settings which are less densely populated than European countries. In addition, some feel internal markets may not be consistent with our nation-wide values.

"We suspect that investigation of the best [allocation] models will consume the attention of health planners for the next decade. Perhaps the highest value, then, will be flexibility, so that modifications can be made as the inevitable problems arise." (Deber et al., 1997)

It is premature to come out in favour of any one form of allocation mechanism. In most cases, it is too early to tell what the results have been, and it is not clear whether there are additional costs associated with creating a more competitive environment. The *Canada Health Act* provides considerable latitude to reform funding mechanisms. Therefore there are no impediments at the national level.

The public should expect to see continuous change and experimentation in this area over the coming years. By and large, these changes should improve the efficiency and quality of health services, provided that the system retains its single-payer, publicly financed character.

The Working Group on Striking a Balance therefore, considers that the advice regarding cash transfers, given by the Forum to the federal government in March, 1996, is still relevant. The Forum recommended that federal government contributions be stable and predictable by establishing the CHST cash floor at the 1997-98 level of $12.5 billion. In providing this advice we were conscious of the fact that there is indeed no magic number. The Working Group further recommends:

a) *That the federal government catalyze reform toward more integrated services in Canada's health care system with a transition fund to support evidence-based projects. The transition fund would support:*

— *pilot projects which have a research and evaluation component, as well as the evaluation dimension of projects already underway;*

— *publication and dissemination of evaluation results;*

— *promotion of suitable models (as shown through evaluation) to interested parties and other jurisdictions; and*

— *emphasis on pilot projects and evaluation of projects to meet the unique needs of aboriginal communities in Canada.*

b) *That, while jurisdictions may approach primary care reform in different ways, key characteristics of pilot projects and reforms should include:*

— *population-based funding for a broad array of preventive, diagnostic and treatment services at the level of primary care;*

— *safeguards to ensure that primary care continues to be provided to those whose conditions result in higher-than-average costs;*

— *multidisciplinary teams of providers (e.g., physicians, nurses, pharmacists); and*

— *delineation of the population served through a variety of approaches (e.g., residence, consumer choice, social or other affiliation).*

c) *That the Conference of Federal/Provincial/ Territorial Deputy Ministers of Health agree to a common evaluation framework to allow provinces to evaluate and compare the results of regionalization initiatives between jurisdictions.*

d) *For provinces which have opted for a regionalized model, that funding and decision making become more integrated at the regional level, particularly in the case of those services which have typically been left out, namely physician services, drugs (and possibly others such as public and mental health services).*

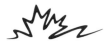

The Public/Private Balance Within the Health Sector

The Working Group on Striking a Balance has given the public/private dimension considerable attention over the course of the last 18 months, because we firmly believe that failure to address this dimension appropriately can frustrate rebalancing efforts in the other two dimensions. On the one hand, there is a misguided public perception, in large part fed by interest groups, self-professed experts and the media, that the only way to reform our health care system is to shift significantly the public/private balance toward more private financing. Our September 1995 discussion paper was in large part meant to address these perceptions and frame the debate more appropriately. However, we realize that beliefs and attitudes change very slowly, particularly when they are grounded in ideology. As governments pursue their efforts to reform and rationalize the system, it is critical to recognize that there is an undefined threshold below which a majority of individuals will see more private funding as part of the solution.

In our view, the Canada Health Act *has been, and continues to be, an effective mechanism to preserve integrity of Canada's publicly financed health care system.*

Reinforcing the role of public financing

As alluded to earlier, our review of public and private financing issues indicates that public funding for medically required health services is undeniably superior to private financing, both from an efficiency and equity perspective (Deber et al., 1997). Private financing tends to promote system fragmentation, cost-shifting and access to services based on ability to pay. Public financing promotes system integrity, cost-control and access based on need.

The vast majority of participants in the Forum's discussion groups expressed overwhelming support for a publicly funded national health care system in accordance with the principles of the *Canada Health Act*. Those who do support more private financing do so because they feel that public funding is inadequate. User fees were largely denounced as a means of financing the system. There was, however, general support among participants nationwide for the right of patients to purchase treatments privately that are not considered medically necessary.

Stakeholders felt that the current balance of public and private financing is sub-optimal, and that the public level may be getting too low to ensure quality and accessibility. They identified a number of issues which need to be addressed, including the definition of comprehensiveness (what's in and what's out) based on evidence, the incentives to shift costs from public to private sources and defining the quality of services which Canadians can expect from medicare. Some participants also warned of the irreversibility of increased private funding.

In our view, the *Canada Health Act* has been, and continues to be, an effective mechanism to preserve integrity of Canada's publicly financed health care system. Physician and hospital services are not in the process of being privatized. National health expenditure accounts have recorded a surge in private funding in a few areas, but this should not necessarily be interpreted as privatization (passive or otherwise) of our health care system. Furthermore, the principles of full public coverage for medically necessary services with no opting-out by taxpayers, and no extra-billing by providers in any form, provide the best recipe to maintain a high degree of publicly supported medicare. No additional safeguards are required at this time for physician and hospital services, provided that the provisions of the *Canada Health Act* are enforced.

Nonetheless, our consultations reveal that the public is concerned about privatization. Most discussion about privatization is based on an emotional and emphatic rejection of the American health system, but we are nowhere near the levels of private financing that characterize the American system. We acknowledge these concerns but we can't emphasize enough that moving toward *private financing* raises issues on a completely different level than moving toward *private delivery* in a publicly funded environment.

At the present time private delivery issues are being decided at the institutional level. Administrators country-wide, as far as we can tell, have incorporated appropriate regulatory provisions when it has been decided that for-profit and/or not-for-profit contractual delivery is a more effective means of delivering services. The role of for-profit financiers is largely limited to drug and dental plans, and out-of-country coverage. People feel ardently that private individuals and corporations should not be "profiting off the backs" of the

sick and needy. There is some tolerance for the profit motive in supplying inputs to the care process (e.g., drugs, devices, ancillary services) but not for comprehensive packages of care.

While this issue is not critical just now, we do have some concerns about the public/private funding split in certain areas of the health system because a significant part of what can reasonably be defined as "medically necessary" has moved outside the realm of physician and hospital services. Data on the public/private split in Canada show a very high concentration of public funding for physician services (99:1) and hospital services (90:1). The funding split for "other institutions" is 70:30, 50:50 for prescription drugs, and 15:85 for "other professionals". If the objective of public insurance for all medically required services is adhered to, additional public funds would have to be generated (offset by an equivalent decline in private outlays) to provide coverage for prescription drugs and probably some of what is included in the "other professionals" category.

The recommendation of the Forum (NFOH. "Directions for Pharmaceutical Policy", 1997) is to aim for full public funding for prescription drugs. In the interim, the pharmaceutical paper recommends the participation of federal and provincial governments, providers and other payers to manage the relationship between public and private plans. An incremental approach is called for to ensure that systems and policies are in place to control costs, improve prescribing, and manage utilization, as well as to take into account the availability of fiscal resources.

The view of the Working Group is that the rate of increase in public spending for home care also merits special attention. On the public side, total spending across all provinces and territories approximated $1.2 billion in 1993-94, and was projected to rise significantly.[10] We don't know what Canadians are spending out-of-pocket for home care, nor do we know to what extent private home care agencies are paid for by third-party insurance. Despite the emphasis on the shift from institutional to community care, no systems are in place to tell us what is being spent, what services are being provided and what the quality of care is like.

Despite the emphasis on the shift from institutional to community care, no systems are in place to tell us what is being spent, what services are being provided and what the quality of care is like.

Continuing care services should be designed to provide more appropriate care in suitable settings. With a rising elderly population, the cost of care is an important consideration. A number of people suggested experimenting with a variety of long term care arrangements ranging from group housing to hotel accommodation in circumstances, for example, where 24 hour supervision is required, however with less medical attention than hospitals provide. Despite willingness to witness experimentation and flexibility in the organizational framework, transfer of care-giving responsibility to families and relatives is only possible if families and relatives are willing, and are provided with substantial support services and supplies.

In response to these observations and concerns, the Working Group is convinced that integrating continuing care services with other care is heading in the right direction. Community-based organizations can then decide upon the right mix and suitable organization of long-term care, and home services, based on locally-determined needs assessments and the values characteristic of each community.

Support for the community health approach is widespread. As we proceed toward integrated services and population-based funding approaches, care for patients and funding for patient care outside the hospital will gradually incorporate continuing care services and supplies, as long as the structures and incentives are aligned to address patient needs. "Fund the care, not the institution," was repeated by consultation participants across the country.

Continuing care services, therefore, should be adequately funded and made available to the public on similar terms and conditions. Given the current fiscal situation, the ability for governments to embark on wide scale reform is limited. The direction, over time, is to provide a smooth transition for patients through the system by funding professional services, medical supplies, home-making and attendant care, and maintenance and preventive care.[11] Without public funding, devolving responsibility to communities and/or regionally-based health care organizations will not be politically or administratively possible.

In the interim, pilot projects are underway, and provinces are experimenting with a variety of models. It is the view of the Working Group that national stewardship is required, particularly for home care and other forms of community care and drug policy; related services and supplies should be considered integral components of publicly funded health services. In these areas, provincial budgets may shrink as total national costs continue to rise. Our priority is total costs versus government preoccupation with their own costs. System incentives, therefore, must ensure that patients are treated in the most appropriate, cost-effective setting, taking into account total public and private costs, both in financial terms and in terms of the burden on care givers, many of whom are women, and often elderly women.

The Working Group on Striking a Balance therefore recommends:

a) *Given the high degree of flexibility in the* **Canada Health Act** *with regard to the organization and delivery of health services, that the federal government not open the* **Canada Health Act.** *Priority should be given to using other policy and legislative instruments to achieve intended goals.*

b) *That federal and provincial governments expand universal public coverage for medically necessary services to encompass prescription drugs, but only after effective cost and utilization control mechanisms have been developed to ensure governments will not incur undue fiscal hardships as a result of the expanded coverage.*

c) *That home care and other forms of community-based care should be considered an integral part of publicly funded health services. Provinces and territories should put in place a proper combination*

of insured services and other mechanisms to meet the needs of post-acute, chronic care, and palliative care patients, and those who, without maintenance and preventive care, would be at risk for reduced quality of life and subsequent institutionalization. A public, single point of entry, as exists in many provinces, should be used to conduct comprehensive multi-disciplinary assessments to determine which services are needed on a case-by-case basis, and to match these services with public and/or private providers.

Improving access to health services

Access to medically required health services based on need rather than ability to pay is the cornerstone of Canada's health care system. Guaranteed payment for insured health services under the *Canada Health Act* clears the most formidable barrier of all, and Canadians take pride in the societal accomplishment this represents.

Nonetheless, universal health care does not resolve all access issues. First, there are distribution problems — urban areas often have an oversupply of resources and rural areas an undersupply. Then, there are general shortages of resources, such as a lack of physicians trained in a particular specialty or a lack of providers to respond to the special needs of certain population groups (e.g., multicultural populations). Third, there are waiting lists for certain services, particularly for specialists and some surgical procedures. These are not issues that can be dealt with by standard-setting and enforcement. Rather, we must ensure that

Canadians retain access to high-quality health services through improvements in the management of health care services.

Those who wish to undermine Medicare often point to waiting lists as proof of its inability to serve all of the people all of the time at a level they find satisfactory. The truth is that most waiting lists for elective surgery are unstructured, many are padded, few are standardized, and even fewer are evaluated. They are therefore quite meaningless. The public, and physicians in particular, tend to blame waiting lists on a lack of resources. However, international comparisons show that the Canadian system is well within the average of OECD countries in terms of the number of practising physicians per 1,000 population, the number of inpatient beds per 1,000 population, and indeed on the high end of expenditures on health per capita.

The truth is that most waiting lists for elective surgery are unstructured, many are padded, few are standardized, and even fewer are evaluated.

An Angus Reid survey commissioned by the Canadian Medical Association (CMA) in 1996, found that 54 percent of respondents reported an increase in waiting times in hospital emergency rooms; 53 percent reported an increase in waiting times for surgery; 43 percent reported longer waiting times for tests such as magnetic resonance imaging (MRI); 41 percent reported a decrease in access to specialist services; 14 percent reported that access to services from their family doctor had worsened; and 25 percent reported

a worsening in the availability of home care services. These are all, however, relative measures — an "increase" in this, a "decrease" in that. More instructive of the level of satisfaction with health service availability in Canada is the 1994-95 National Population Health Survey which recorded that 96 percent of 50,000 people asked, felt they had reasonable access to needed health care services. Where waiting in the queue can cause serious problems, the system generally does a good job of ensuring that patients are served fairly.

The Fraser Institute periodically surveys waiting times for specialist physicians representing 10 different medical specialties across the country. The survey covers the length of time consumers wait for services, and the numbers of persons on waiting lists in each of the provinces. Its findings show considerable variation in waiting times. Following the same research agenda, the College of Family Physicians of Canada, in 1996, surveyed its members on quality of care issues. Nine out of 10 family physicians expressed concern that waiting lists were becoming the norm. Most family physicians (86 percent) reported that delays and difficulties getting access to health care had put, or were putting, their patients at risk. As well, 82 percent of family physicians reported spending more time than they did five years ago trying to get access to health care services for their patients. Most family physicians cited longer waiting lists at each stage of patient care: 79 percent stated that waiting times for specialists were longer; 78 percent reported that waits for hospital admissions were longer; 72 percent pointed to longer waiting times for diagnostic testing; and 62 percent reported having problems with community-based health services once their patients were discharged.

No doubt some people wait too long, and this group's stories are retailed as evidence that the system does not and cannot work. We hear much less about the opposite side of the coin: unnecessary surgery and people being served ahead of those with far greater problems. Experience in Canada (e.g., coronary surgery prioritization in Ontario), and abroad (e.g., reduction of waiting lists in Sweden in the early 1990s) suggests that public health care systems can reduce waiting lists without increasing spending. The key is to ensure that waiting lists are structured and prioritized, and that incentives are in place to ensure that patients are served before their risk, or their degree of suffering becomes unacceptably high. The solution is management, monitoring, and evaluation—not a bewildering and expensive array of public and private alternatives. If ability to pay becomes the key factor in obtaining better access, the whole premise of Medicare is violated.

Tied in with the focus on better management, the Evidence-Based Decision Making Working Group has recommended the development of a nation-wide health information system. The Striking a Balance Working Group views this recommendation as an opportunity to enhance access, not only to information, but to quality services. New technologies are coming on the market, and a system-wide effort is required to assess and integrate them when they are proven to be the best available treatment alternative. Based on what the consumers of health services have told the Forum, total quality management (TQM) is a consideration as vital to the health sector as to manufacturing. A set of core quality indicators must be determined that will serve as benchmarks against which the public can hold provincial administrators and decision makers accountable.

It is likely that information systems will advance to the point where some of the particularly vexing challenges in Canada — equitable geographic distribution and multicultural/multilingual accessibility — can be improved by the integration of existing technology. The *Economist* (1994) reports that development continues in the processing and transferring of complex pieces of information, including X-rays, or even moving pictures of a surgical operation, by satellites or fibre-optic cable. Technology has already advanced to a stage where an individual can personally determine information about her health status with home test kits for pregnancy. Soon, there will be devices that can determine the chemical content of blood simply by touching the skin. These technological advances will broaden access to information that throughout history has been the purview of medical professionals. But technology should not be adopted blindly. At every stage, technological initiatives should be measured against the principles of universal and equitable access, social values and privacy/confidentiality considerations.

The Working Group on Striking a Balance therefore recommends:

That provincial/territorial agencies together with a national agency (NFOH, Evidence, 1997), give priority to developing a set of indicators and benchmarks to be used by all jurisdictions for assessment of the state of access to appropriate health services, and as part of their public reporting function, collect and make this information public at regular intervals.

Defining medically necessary services: holy grail or red herring?

Publicly funded health care in Canada has incorporated the concept of "medically necessary services" as a central feature of insured services, enshrined in the vocabulary of the *Canada Health Act*. The Act requires public insurance of hospital and medically necessary physician services but does not require public funding of anything else. Attempts at refining the definition of medical necessity have been prominent features of health care discourse, particularly since the latest wave of health reform. We offer the following observations on the nature and importance of this debate.

First, there has always been a distinction between the logical and applied meaning of medical necessity. Logically, a medically nec-

The service in itself is neither medically necessary or unnecessary; necessity is linked to the nature of the condition for which it is prescribed.

essary service is one that is required to address legitimate medical needs. The service in itself is neither medically necessary or unnecessary; necessity is linked to the nature of the condition for which it is prescribed. A service that is medically necessary in most instances may be entirely useless in some. Conversely, a service that is by and large ineffective may be highly effective in a few instances.

In practice, the health care system has defined services as either medically necessary or not to identify which services will be paid for by the public purse, and which will be left to private insurance of individual consumers. This has two predictable consequences: the public system will pay for some services that are inefficiently or ineffectively deployed, while other potentially very useful and — on the grounds of common sense — necessary services will not be publicly funded. This is no mystery either to health care practitioners or system managers and designers. To date it has been considered the only easily understood, and simple-to-administer way to distinguish between necessary and unnecessary services, despite its adverse consequences. It is imperfect, but better than any known alternative.

Because of the problems created by this arbitrary set of distinctions, a number of people have tried to develop schemes to define the circumstances that would trigger public funding as opposed to including or excluding services *in toto* (Deber et al., 1997). These attempts are often creative and well intentioned, but we have not come across any that solves the problem efficiently. To implement a system with several decision rules or junctures would require cumbersome procedures and a complex series of judgments. In the end, it appears that these schemes would require an enormous amount of effort to reduce but not eliminate the capriciousness of the current in-or-out system.[12]

Second, there is a great deal of discussion about the consequences of de-insurance of services and their impact on medicare. While it is true that a number of provinces have wholly or partially de-insured a number of services previously covered by public funding, these actions are not a threat to medicare *per se*. Medicare was originally intended to cover hospital and doctor services, and by law it continues to do so today. Many governments chose to expand the scope of medicare by insuring services previously left to private funding and/or third-party insurance in the 1970s and early 1980s. Now they are clawing back this expansion.

The core elements are just as firmly enshrined in law and practice as they were decades ago. This is not to say that the recent wave of de-insurance is not without consequences. When services are covered through public funding, the income effect is progressive: poor people benefit disproportionately from a shift from private payment to public funding. Similarly, when services are de-insured, by and large the effect is regressive: both wealthy and poor people (other than the indigent insured by other means) pay the same amount for previously funded public services, which is a greater hardship for the poor. Aside from the regressiveness of de-insurance, the other main consequence is to reveal yet again the arbitrariness of the definition of medical necessity.

For it is clear that many recently de-insured services are medically necessary by any common-sense definition, for example, optometric care for people with eyesight problems.

Third, while the term "health insurance" is coupled with medicare, the publicly funded system does not really operate like an insurance scheme. Most insurance involves the pooling of risk in a population, all of whom hope never to experience the event that triggers a payout. Health care is different. It is expected that the population will use the services at regular intervals, and the service use is, in many cases, not a sign of a catastrophic or unwelcome bit of bad luck, but as an important and positive universal service. Medicare covers services that are in this sense more analogous to highways — public goods whose use enhances quality of life, wealth, etc.

Fourth, even within the narrow definition of medical necessity as enshrined in the *Canada Health Act,* the system has expansionist tendencies. Doctors and hospitals can do many more things than they could 30 years ago. Hospitals are involved in a much wider range of diagnostic and therapeutic activities, even while average length of stay declines persistently. Doctors have a more sophisticated diagnostic and therapeutic arsenal (laboratory tests, pharmaceuticals) at their disposal. The overall capacity of the system expanded tremendously in the decade and a half following national medicare, and the system has until recently continued to absorb large numbers of new physicians despite a slow-growing population and apparent improvements in overall health status of the population (e.g., increased life expectancy, reduced incidence of debilitating conditions such as stroke). Therefore, restricting the definition of medical necessity to hospitals and doctors does not necessarily mean restricting the range of services to which the public has access as a matter of entitlement.

We do not foresee a redefinition of medical necessity that would clearly yield more benefits than costs.

An unintended consequence of the *Canada Health Act* definition of medical necessity is an incentive to provide services either in hospital or by a physician to guarantee publicly funded status. This is another problem with the arbitrary definition: a preference emerges for inefficient deployment of resources in order to "play the game" mandated by the *Canada Health Act.*

Fifth, many of the problems associated with the definition of medical necessity arise from the traditional fee-for-service reimbursement mechanisms for physicians. When the state pays for services on an itemized basis, it is essential to define which items are reimbursable and which are not. The judgment about whether something is medically necessary in the end has very little to do with its anticipated health benefit *per se*. It has everything to do with whether physicians are paid for their efforts. Similarly, paying hospitals to provide a certain amount of care or number of patient-days guarantees a preference for hospital use when funding and governance of health programs are fragmented, with autonomous boards and unco-ordinated delivery mechanisms.

We do not foresee a redefinition of medical necessity that would clearly yield more benefits than costs (Charles et al., 1996). Health science is remarkably productive, and new ways to diagnose and treat disease emerge with great speed on a number of fronts. Any list-based approach to defining medical necessity — with some things publicly funded and others not — will invariably be valid for only a short period of time due to the pace of technological change. Any list-based approach will carry with it the defects of its forebears, namely, the almost invariably flawed assumption that any service is either always useful or always useless (Hurley et al., 1996). The alternatives — attempting to define the circumstances under which a service is useful or not — have thus far been plagued with complexity while failing to solve the conceptual problems. One also has to question what role is left for professional judgment if insured services could be defined in such a precise, objective manner.

That doesn't mean we shouldn't be thinking about what blocks of services the public system should cover. To reiterate, services should be provided when necessary, and the system should incorporate in a rational way, those services for which there is a medical need. There are clear signals that the organization and delivery of services will change substantially. Regionalization is sweeping the country, and the common theme is unified governance and administration combined with global funding and flexible allocation of resources. In theory at least, these developments remove the pressure to define medical necessity precisely and arbitrarily. A regional board, for example, could be given a certain amount of money per person, and be allowed to judge where the resources should be deployed most effectively to achieve its goals (assuming the maintenance of basic standards of safety and effectiveness and a reasonable amount of uniformity in the system). Significantly, medical care and reimbursement remain outside the regional structures to date, but there are many (including this Working Group) who believe their incorporation is inevitable and desirable.

Similarly, there is widespread interest in primary care reform. Should fee-for-service as the primary reimbursement mechanism disappear or undergo substantial modification, the need for precise definitions of which services merit public coverage diminishes substantially. A primary health centre model with integrated services and population based funding permits, in theory, the most efficient use of labour by decoupling payment and delivery (i.e. it is no longer a matter of the physician providing the service to obtain payment).

If these trends persist, in our view the medical necessity definition issue will no longer be as prominent as it is now. There will certainly be debates about the effectiveness of services and criteria for determining whether provision is efficient. The above-cited changes would cast resource allocation dilemmas in a different form rather than eliminate them entirely. The insistence on greater accountability, and resource deployment and outcome measurement based on value for money, require evaluation techniques and information systems that are just developing. But all these trends should allow the system to move away from rigid and arbitrary definitions.

In the meantime, we could do a lot worse than maintaining the *Canada Health Act* status quo, despite its problems. These legally enshrined provisions are a buffer against the repeated calls for privatization and the creation of a multi-tiered system. The status quo also ensures that debates about what is covered and what is not remain in the public and political realm. If the public are dissatisfied with government decisions about de-insurance or failure to expand coverage to certain areas, they can exercise their judgment at the ballot box and through the usual channels of political discourse. Regionalization creates authoritative and, in some cases, publicly elected bodies which can add their voices to the discussion and debate. The challenge will be to combine articulated values with an evidence-based approach to determine which services should be publicly funded and which should not on grounds unrelated to individual payments. This is no small challenge, but it is a different challenge and redefines the issue substantially.

The Working Group on Striking a Balance therefore recommends:

That adoption of a detailed list of medically necessary services (core services) should be resisted by all jurisdictions. A flexible definition of "medical necessity" which incorporates the concepts of evidence, appropriateness and effectiveness of services, however, may be useful in some jurisdictions.

Conclusion

In preparing this report, we recognize that much of what we have to say about striking a balance rests on the need to understand the world a certain way, in contrast to taking specific and direct action. If our audience accepts this view, then we will have accomplished a significant part of our mandate.

In our specific recommendations, we have avoided the temptation of dictating in detail or by what magnitude the balance of resources should shift. Rather, we have commented on the need to articulate clearly the broad values and principles at play, the need to improve the use and availability of information and evidence, and the need to align decision-making structures and incentives properly within and outside the health sector. In the final analysis, we must have faith in the ability of governments, health services providers and individuals to make the right choices.

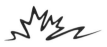

Endnotes

1. These are: British Columbia — *Closer to Home* (1991), Alberta — The *Rainbow Report: Our Vision for Health* (1989), Saskatchewan — *Future Directions for Health Care in Saskatchewan* (1990), Ontario — *Towards a Shared Direction for Health in Ontario* (1987) and *Deciding the Future of Our Health Care* (1989), Quebec — *Commission d'enquête sur les services de santé et les services sociaux* (1988), New Brunswick — *Report of the Commission on Selected Health Care Programs* (1989) and Nova Scotia — *Towards a New Strategy* (1989).

2. Purchasing power parity equalizes dollar prices in every country so that cross-country comparisons reflect real-value comparisons. Dollar values (representing purchasing power parity) are obtained by special conversion factors designed to equalize the purchasing power (quantities of goods and services that can be purchased for a dollar) of currencies in respective countries.

3. We recognize that life cannot be reduced to a data set on expenditures. Furthermore, GDP does not capture the totality of economic activity in society, particularly in the informal/voluntary sector. However, GDP is a relatively well-established indicator, comparable within and outside Canada. This approach is the simplest and most straightforward way to explain our mandate and set forth our recommendations.

4. National Health Expenditures in Canada, 1975-94, User's Guide, p. 9. Note that in practice, hospitals may choose to cross-subsidize medically necessary procedures with funding raised through these private sources. One possible explanation for the increase in "private" hospital expenditures may lie in attempts by hospitals to cushion the blow of budget reductions by generating private revenue.

5. There are exceptions. Because of limited supply, recipients of organ transplants are usually determined on an ability-to-benefit basis.

6. In 1994, real total health expenditures (in 1986 dollars) were $2,109 per capita in Alberta and $2,016 per capita in Ontario. The provincial average for real total health expenditures (1986 dollars) was $1,875. The situation may have changed from 1994 to the present.

7. See F/P/T Advisory Committee's report, *The Victoria Report on Physician Remuneration: A model for the reorganization of primary care and the introduction of population-based funding.*

8. Population-based funding means that provincial funding would be provided to organizations based on the number of people for whom they are accountable (with adjustments for age, sex and other factors). Organizations would then be free to remunerate physicians and other providers by fee-for-service, salary, capitation or any combination thereof.

9. Leibovich, Bergman and Béland (1997) discuss the need for an integrated system of care for the frail elderly.

10. Verbal communication (October, 1996) with Evelyn Shapiro, (Senior Researcher at the Manitoba Centre for Health Policy and Evaluation), in relation to provincial responses to survey questions posed by the Manitoba Centre.

11. A precise definition of what should be covered under 'home care' carries with it the same complexity as defining what is medically necessary (see section, 'Defining medically necessary services: holy grail or red herring?'- p. 40).

12. Appeal processes and exception boards exist in all provinces.

References

Alberta. *The Rainbow Report: Our Vision for Health*. Edmonton: Premier's Commission on Future Health Care for Albertans, 1989.

Alberta Health. *Home Care Client Classification (HCCC) System Final Report*, March 1994.

Angus, Doug E. *Review of significant health care commissions and task forces in Canada since 1983-84*. Ottawa: Canadian Hospital Association, 1991.

Angus, Doug E., Ludwig Auer, J. Eden Cloutier, and Terry Albert. *Sustainable Health Care for Canada*. Ottawa: Queens University/University of Ottawa, 1995.

Angus Reid Group Inc. Presentation to the National Forum on Health (October, 1994).

Arweiler, Delphine. "International Comparisons of Health Expenditures." International Comparison Series Paper. *Papers Commissioned by the National Forum on Health*. Ottawa, 1997 (in press).

Arweiler, Delphine. "Price and quantity." Commissioned by the National Forum on Health, 1996.

British Columbia. *Closer to Home: the Report of the British Columbia Health Care Programs on Health Care and Costs*. Victoria: Crown Publications, 1991.

Brousselle, Astrid. "Controlling Health Care Costs: What Matters." International Comparison Series Paper. *Papers Commissioned by the National Forum on Health*. Ottawa, 1997 (in press).

Brownwell, M., and N. Roos. *Monitoring the Winnipeg Hospital System: the Update Report and Summary, 1993/94*. Manitoba Centre for Health Policy and Evaluation, January 1996.

Canada. Health Canada. *Financial Incentives in the Canadian Health System*. Series of reports by investigators at the Centre for Health Economics and Policy Analysis, M.Giacomini, principal investigator. Ottawa, 1996.

_____. *National Health Expenditures in Canada: 1975-94*. Ottawa, 1996.

_____. Health and Welfare Canada. *Achieving Health For All: A Framework for Health Promotion*. (Epp Report) Ottawa, 1986.

_____. *A New Perspective on the Health of Canadians*. (Lalonde Report). Ottawa, 1974.

_____. National Forum on Health. *Maintaining a National Health Care System:*

A Question of Principle(s) ... and Money. Ottawa, 1996.

_____. "Creating a Culture of Evidence-Based Decision Making - Synthesis Report." *Canada Health Action: Building on the Legacy* Vol. II. Ottawa, 1997.

_____. "Determinants of Health Working Group Synthesis Report." *Canada Health Action: Building on the Legacy.* Volume II. Ottawa, 1997.

_____. "Directions for Pharmaceutical Policy in Canada." *Canada Health Action: Building on the Legacy.* Vol. II. Ottawa, 1997.

_____. "Values Working Group Synthesis Report." *Canada Health Action: Building on the Legacy.* Vol. II. Ottawa, 1997.

_____. *The Public and Private Financing of Canada's Health System.* Ottawa, 1995.

_____. Statistics Canada. *National Population Health Survey.* Ottawa, 1994-95.

Canadian Medical Association. *The Future of Health and Health Care in Canada.* Briefing document for the 129th Meeting of the General Council of the CMA, 1996.

Centre for International Statistics at the Canadian Council for Social Development. "Health Spending and Health Status: An International Comparison." International Comparison Series Paper. *Papers Commissioned by the National Forum on Health.* Ottawa, 1997 (in press).

Charles, C.A., J. Lomas, M. Giacomini, V. Bhatia, and V. Vincent. *The Role of Medical Necessity in Canadian Health Policy: Four Meanings and . . . A Funeral?* Centre for Health Economics & Policy Analysis, Working Paper 96-18. McMaster University, 1996.

Contandriopoulos, André-Pierre, François Champagne, Jean-Louis Denis, Claude Sicotte, Anne Lemay, Delphine Arweiler, Marc-André Fournier, Daniel Reinharz, and Louise-Hélène Trottier. *Financial Incentives/Disincentives in Canada's Health System.* Gris-Université de Montréal, Groupe SECOR, March 1996.

Deber, Raisa, Lutchmie Narine, Pat Baranek, Natasha Hilfer, Katya Masnyk Duvalko, Randi Zlotnik-Shaul, Peter Coyte, George Pink, and A. Paul Williams. "The Public/Private Mix in Canada's Health System." *Papers Commissioned by the National Forum on Health.* Ottawa, 1997 (in press).

Deber, R., and B. Swan. "Puzzling Issues in Health Care Financing." International Comparison Series Paper. *Papers Commissioned by the National Forum on Health.* Ottawa, 1997 (in press).

DeCoster, C., Sandra Peterson, and Paul Kasian. *Alternatives to Acute Care*. Manitoba Centre for Health Policy and Evaluation, 1996.

Economist. *The Economist Survey of the Future of Medicine: Peering into 2010*. March 19, 1994.

Ekos Research Associates Inc. *Rethinking Government 95-1*. Ottawa, 1995.

Evans, R.G. "Going for the Gold: The Redistributive Agenda Behind Market-Based Health Care Reform." *Journal of Health Politics, Policy and Law*, April, 1997 (in press).

_____. *Squaring the Circle: Reconciling Fee for Service with Global Expenditure Control*. Health Policy Research Unit Discussion Paper HPRU 88: 8D, Division of Health Services Research and Development. Vancouver: University of British Columbia, 1988.

Evans, R.G., Morris L. Barer, and Theodore R. Marmor, eds. *Why Are Some People Healthy and Others Not? The Determinants of Health of Populations*. New York: Walter de Gruyter, 1994.

Federal/Provincial/Territorial Advisory Committee on Health Services. *Victoria Report on Physician Remuneration: A model for the reorganization of primary care and the introduction of population-based funding*, 1995.

Federal/Provincial/Territorial Advisory Committee on Population Health. *Strategies for Population Health: Investing in the Health of Canadians*. Report prepared for the meeting of the Ministers of Health, Halifax, Nova Scotia, September 14-15, 1994.

Federal/Provincial/Territorial Deputy Ministers of Health paper prepared by the Working Group on Health Services Utilization. *When Less Is Better: Using Canada's Hospitals Efficiently*, June 1994.

Fournier, M.A. "The Impact of Health Care Infrastructures and Human Resources Characteristics on Health Expenditures." International Comparison Series Paper. *Papers Commissioned by the National Forum on Health*. Ottawa, 1997 (in press).

Fraser Institute. *Waiting your turn: hospital waiting lists in Canada*. Vancouver, 1995.

Groupe de Recherche Interdisciplinaire en Santé (GRIS) "How Canada's Health Care System Compares with that of Other Countries - An overview." International Comparison Series Paper. *Papers Commissioned by the National Forum on Health*. Ottawa, 1997 (in press).

Health Services Utilization and Research Commission. *Barriers to Community Care: Final Report*. Saskatoon, 1994.

Hurley, Jeremiah, Stephen Birch, Greg Stoddart, George Torrance and Victoria Vincent. *Defying Definition: Medical Necessity and Health Policy Making*. Centre for Health Economics and Policy Analysis, McMaster University, 1996.

Kennedy, W. "Managing Pharmaceutical Expenditures: How Canada Compares." International Comparison Series Paper. *Papers Commissioned by the National Forum on Health*. Ottawa, 1997 (in press).

Leibovich, E., H. Bergman, and F. Béland. "Health Care Expenditures and the Aging Population in Canada." International Comparison Series Paper. *Papers Commissioned by the National Forum on Health*. Ottawa, 1997 (in press).

Lewis, Steven. *Sickness Care, Health and Well-Being: Breaking the Continuum and Implications for the Hospital of the Future*. Paper presented at conference on the 'Hospital of Tomorrow: What Role Will It Play?' Montréal, October 4, 1996.

Marriott, J., and A. Mable. "Integrated Models: International Trends and Implications for Canada." International Comparison Series Paper. *Papers Commissioned by the National Forum on Health*. Ottawa, 1997 (in press).

Maslove, A. *National Goals and the Federal Role in Health Care*. National Forum on Health: Ottawa, 1996.

Matre S., and R. Deber. "From Equal Access to Health Care to Equitable Access to Health: A Review of Canadian Provincial Health Commissions and Report." *International Journal of Health Services*, 22. 4 (1992).

Morgan, S. "Issues for Canadian Pharmaceutical Policy." *Papers Commissioned by the National Forum on Health*. Ottawa, 1997 (in press).

New Brunswick. Health and Community Services. *Evaluation Report of the Single Entry Point Pilot Project*. Bureau de Consultation Evaco enr., April 1991.

New Brunswick. *Report of the Commission on Selected Health Care Programs*. Fredericton: Commission on Selecte Health Care Programs, 1989.

Nova Scotia. *The Report of the Nova Scotia Royal Commission on Health Care: Towards a New Strategy*. Halifax: Royal Commission on Health Care, 1989.

OECD. *The Reform of Health Care Systems: A Review of 17 OECD Countries*. Paris, 1994.

OECD. Health Data 1996. Paris, 1996.

Ontario. *Toward a shared direction for health in Ontario: report of the Ontario Health Review Panel*. Toronto: Health Review Panel, 1987.

_____. Ministry of Health. *Deciding the future of our health care: an overview of areas for public discussion:* Toronto: Queen's Printer, 1989.

Pearson, Lester B. *Medicare and Health Services: The Federal Government's Role.* Statements by the Right Honourable L.B. Pearson, Prime Minister of Canada, at the Federal-Provincial Conference, Ottawa, July 19-20, 1965.

Pew Health Professions Commission. *Critical Challenges: Revitalizing the Health Profession for the 21st Century.* San Francisco, CA: UCSF Center for the Health Professions, 1995.

Québec. Commission d'enquête sur les services de santé et les services sociaux. *Rapport de la commission d'enquête sur les services de santé et les services sociaux.* Québec : Publications de Québec, 1988.

Saskatchewan. *Future directions for health care in Saskatchewan.* Regina: Saskatchewan Commission on Directions in Health Care, 1990.

Scott, G. "International Comparison of the Hospital Sector." International Comparison Series Paper. *Papers Commissioned by the National Forum on Health.* Ottawa, 1997 (in press).

Stoddart, Greg L. *The Challenge of Producing Health in Modern Economies. CIAR Program in Population Health,* Working Paper No. 46, The Canadian Institute for Advanced Research, 1995.

Sullivan, Terrence. "Commentary on Health Care Expenditures, Social Spending and Health Status." International Comparison Series Paper. *Papers Commissioned by the National Forum on Health.* Ottawa, 1997 (in press).

World Health Organization International Conference on Health Promotion, Health Canada, and the Canadian Public Health Association. *Ottawa Charter on Health Promotion,* 1986.

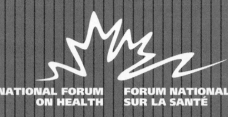

NATIONAL FORUM
ON HEALTH

FORUM NATIONAL
SUR LA SANTÉ

Determinants
of Health
Working
Group
Synthesis
Report

Determinants of Health Working Group

Marc Renaud, Ph.D. (Chair)
Debbie Good, C.A.
Louise Nadeau, Ph.D.
Judith Ritchie, Ph.D.
Roberta Way-Clark, M.A.

Carmen Connolly (Policy Analyst)

Acknowledgements

As members of the Determinants of Health Working Group, we wish to recognize the contribution and support we received from many people to carry out our work on the determinants of health for the National Forum on Health. We received over 400 nominations from individuals from across the country of potential authors for our background papers. Jack Altman, Nancy Kotani, Irving Rootman, Fernand Turcotte and John Wright served as members of a Review Committee who provided advice on the selection of authors. The authors of the 30 commissioned papers, who are identified at the end of this document, generated a rich source of ideas and challenges. The Working Group was assisted in the synthesis of these papers by Colette Biron, Louise Bouchard, Susan Liley and Miriam Stewart. We are also grateful to the many Canadians who provided advice through the Forum's consultation process that involved discussion groups, conferences, surveys and written submissions. We received assistance from John Evans, Fraser Mustard, Martin Wilk, Michael Wolfson and numerous friends and colleagues with whom we have had the opportunity to debate our ideas. And finally, our fellow Forum members, especially Bill Blundell and Duncan Sinclair who assisted us in our analysis, enriched our work through the many discussions that took place during the Forum's tenure. For this, we say a very warm thank you.

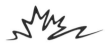

Preface

In the last 50 years, life expectancy in Canada has increased by 15 years. This tremendous improvement, however, is at risk of being compromised by the problems facing our children in this country, the difficulties that communities are experiencing in mobilizing and the high rate of unemployment, especially among youth. Considering the growing evidence on the non–medical determinants of health and on examples of successful interventions, the Working Group believes there is an urgent need for action. It is our legacy in health that is at stake.

Contents

Acknowledgements

Preface

1. Overview 3

    1.1   First Observation: Knowledge of What Makes People Healthy 5

           1.1.1   The Socioeconomic Gradient 5

           1.1.2   Healthy Childhood Development 6

           1.1.3   The Unexplained: Gender Differences 8

    1.2   Second Observation: Beyond Health Care Policies. 9

           1.2.1   Income Distribution 9

           1.2.2   Children and Families 9

           1.2.3   Employment 11

           1.2.4   Strengthening Community Action 12

           1.2.5   The Role of Governments. 12

2. Our Approach 14

3. Key Findings About the Environment 15

    3.1   Employment and the Economy. 15

    3.2   Communities, Families, Schools and Workplaces 16

           3.2.1   Communities that Create Health 17

           3.2.2   Families that Create Health 20

           3.2.3   Schools that Create Health 22

           3.2.4   Workplaces that Create Health 23

4. Key Findings About Vulnerable Groups 24

    4.1   Children's Health 24

    4.2   Youth Health 27

    4.3   Adult Health 31

    4.4   Seniors' Health 34

5. Lessons Learned 37

    5.1   Lessons Learned from Research on the Determinants of Health 38

    5.2   Lessons Learned from Success Stories 39

6. Policy Implications and Recommendations 42

    6.1   Investing in Children 43

            6.1.1   Programs for Children and Families 44

            6.1.2   Income Support Programs 45

    6.2   Communities 47

    6.3   Employment 50

    6.4   Research, Monitoring and Evaluation 51

7. Conclusion 53

Endnotes 56

List of Commissioned Papers 60

1. Overview

Physicians, biochemists, and the general public assume that the body is a machine that can be protected mainly by physical and chemical intervention. This approach, rooted in 17th century science, has led to widespread indifference to the influence of the primary determinants of human health—environment and personal behaviour—and emphasizes the role of medical treatment, which is actually less important than either of the others.

Thomas McKeown, Human Nature, 1(4), April 1978, p. 57.

Since the Second World War, Canadians have seen their life expectancy increase by more than 15 years.[1] This improvement is even more stunning over an extended period: at the beginning of the 19th century, one could not expect to live past 40. A newborn child today may expect to live to be 74 years old if he is male, and 81 if she is female. Today, less than 1 of every 100 children is stillborn, compared to 1 of 3 in the early 1800s and 1 of 10 in the early 1900s. Cemeteries are no longer at the centre of our towns and villages. Good health now typifies our lives.

To what do we owe such remarkable progress in our life expectancy? For years, McKeown and many others argued what is now a known fact: that if health status is improving, it is not necessarily due to the steps taken when we are ill, but rather to the fact that we are not as sick as before. While interventions such as immunization and treatments have a role to play in achieving and maintaining good health, a higher standard of living and a healthier environment are also major factors.

The National Forum on Health has pondered this finding at length and has considered how it fits into public policies as we enter the 21st century. The main question we asked ourselves was; in these times of economic and social hardship, what actions must be taken to allow Canadians to continue to enjoy a long life and, if possible, to increase their health status?

Many health and social indicators are promising—life expectancy has increased while crime, injuries, per capita alcohol intake and smoking among males have decreased. Many people believe, however, that elements in our current economic and social environment put our health at risk. We believe this could contribute to our death at a younger age than the previous generation. Child poverty, unemployment, youth underemployment, involuntary retirement, labour force restructuring, cuts in social programs, decreases in real income, income inequalities, the disintegration of communities as we once knew them and the ever-increasing pressures of work on families could lead to declines rather than increases in life expectancy. We are already starting to see some worrisome signs, such as increases in stress-related diseases and mental health problems associated with unemployment, increases in smoking rates among women, and suicide rates among youth and continuing high rates of low birth weight babies.

In these times of economic and social hardship, what actions must be taken to allow Canadians to continue to enjoy a long life and, if possible, to increase their health status?

We know that societies can improve or worsen their health by influencing the quality of the social environments in which people live and work. The most striking examples of this effect are, on the one hand, in Japan, where in a span of 30 years, life expectancy has increased more than in any other country, and, on the other hand, in Eastern Europe, where there has been a dramatic reduction in life expectancy. Both the improvement and the reduction in life expectancy may be attributable to comparably drastic changes in the social and economic environment.[2]

As the *Report on the Health of Canadians* states,

> Canadians have made good progress in improving their overall level of health, and are currently among the healthiest people in the world. Canadians are living longer, fewer infants are dying in the first year of life, and early deaths due to heart disease and injuries have declined. However, some indicators show a stable or worsening trend, indicating that there is an ongoing need for action to improve our health. ... There are a number of trends that are cause for concern because of their potential impact on the health of Canadians.[3]

There has been a great deal of discussion about the importance of personal health practices for the health of individuals and populations. While we have known for some time that poor health practices (such as smoking, poor eating habits or substance abuse) are determinants of ill health, we know that such practices are very much influenced by the social and economic environments in which people live and work. They involve less of an

individual choice than was once thought.

For example, tobacco is the most worrisome substance used among youth. Young people who lack some of the basic prerequisites of health (such as supportive parents and education) are more likely to smoke and misuse other substances than other adolescents.[4] In 1994, 29% of young women aged 15 to 19 and 28% of young men in the same age range were smokers.[5] The earlier a person becomes addicted, the greater their chances of developing a tobacco–related disease.

The Working Group strongly supports the need to continue to encourage Canadians to adopt positive health practices. At the same time, we have chosen to focus our attention on the broader social and economic factors that influence all of our choices.

It has also been recognized that the physical environment is one of the many types of causal pathways or mechanisms that might lead to the differences in health status that are observed across populations and stages of the life cycle. Differential exposures to physical, chemical and biological agents at home, at work and in the community cause differences in health status.[6,7] The possible effects on health of changes in the physical environment have not been extensively examined and the Forum was not able to pursue work in this area during the course of its mandate and supports further research on the physical environment as a determinant of health.

To identify what can be done to buffer the health impact of changes in the social and economic environment, the Determinants of Health Working Group consulted with top specialists. We asked them to identify the best ways of improving the health of children, youth, adults and seniors and to consider issues related to gender during these life stages. We asked them to provide us with examples of effective measures that could be taken. We said to them, "Show us how education can change people's lives and improve their health. Show us how health and the labour force are connected. Show us how mobilizing a community can benefit people's lives. Show us what a family can do. Show us that national economic policies can make a difference."

The research and consultations led us to two important observations. First, we have come a long way in the last decade in determining what makes people healthy. Second, despite this new knowledge base and the success stories witnessed in many communities, there is still an obsession with health care rather than health. Although we are now beginning to understand what can be done, this understanding is not being followed by concrete action. We have not yet developed health policies, only health care policies. Change is needed.

1.1 First Observation: Knowledge of What Makes People Healthy

1.1.1 The Socioeconomic Gradient

Our first observation is based on the work of the Canadian Institute for Advanced Research[8] and on research in health promotion. Researchers have known for a long time, by studying the relationships between variables, that social factors and health are correlated. It is not news, for instance, that people with high income and education levels tend to be healthier and live longer than people who fall lower on the socioeconomic scale. It has also been known for some time that countries where incomes are more evenly distributed have a healthier population in terms of life expectancy, quality of life and mortality rates. In the last 10 years, we have learned that these correlations are signs of a causal link. We are now certain that there are social, economic and cultural determinants of health, just as genetics and health services are determinants.

We know that the health of the population is a gradient when assessed against measurements like levels of income and education, type of work and degree of social support. The higher one's social status, the better one's health (Figure 1 and 2). The link is more pronounced in more hierarchical countries. This relationship cannot be attributed strictly to reverse causality or to the poor lifestyle choices (e.g., inappropriate alcohol consumption, unhealthy eating, unsafe sex) by people in the bottom part of the gradient (Figure 3). Rather, it seems that the relationship exists for all causes of death, independent of known risk factors[9]. It might be explained by the fact that the higher a person is on the social scale, the better the person's self-esteem, sense of control over one's life and resiliency. (Resiliency is the ability to bounce back into shape and position; or the ability to recover strength and spirits quickly.). In contrast, countries that are more prosperous and where resources are more evenly distributed have a healthier population. The more equal a society, the more widely shared are feelings of self-esteem and control, the more empowered are its members, and the better is overall health status. (Empowerment refers to the idea that in order to further the

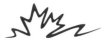

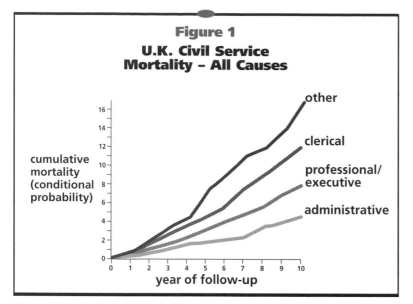

Figure 1

U.K. Civil Service
Mortality – All Causes

cumulative
mortality
(conditional
probability)

other
clerical
professional/
executive
administrative

year of follow-up

Source: The Canadian Institute for Advanced Research

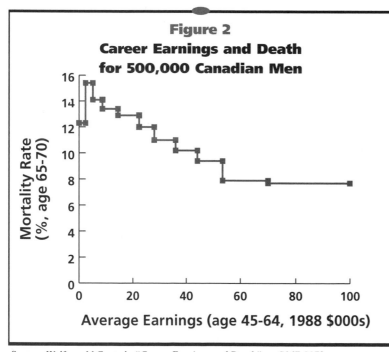

Figure 2

Career Earnings and Death
for 500,000 Canadian Men

Mortality Rate
(%, age 65-70)

Average Earnings (age 45-64, 1988 $000s)

Source: Wolfson, M.C. et al., "Career Earnings and Death", p. S167-S179

FIGURE 2
This figure shows that socioeconomic status (SES)
preceded in time the health consequences. In other
words, the data are highly suggestive that the direction of casualty runs from SES to health status,
rather than the reverse.

FIGURE 1
This figure demonstrates that over a ten–year period,
the mortality rate of male manual (other) and office
workers was three times higher than that of male
professionals and administrative staff. This implies
the existence of a non–specific etiological process
which is correlated with the individual's position in
the hierarchy and which can be expressed through a
variety of illnesses.

democratization process of our societies, we
have to better apportion power, with the likely
effect of improving people's health).

1.1.2 Healthy Childhood Development

An individual's competence and coping style
are largely set during the early period of life
when the brain is most "plastic" or pliable.
How the cortex of the brain develops is of
fundamental importance in understanding how
we cope with the challenges of everyday life
in both work and non-work environments.

Evidence shows that individuals who cope
poorly have a substantial outpouring of hormones into the bloodstream. These hormones,
particularly steroids, can suppress other body
systems such as those that are part of the host
defence system (for example, the immune system); if the hormones stay elevated, they can
weaken an individual's response to the causes
of disease. High steroid levels also affect the
neurons and the functioning of the brain, particularly in the hippocampus. Other chemical
mediators that influence coping are increased
or decreased in response to challenges. Thus,
an individual who does not cope well with the
chronic challenges of everyday life is vulnerable to the early expression of many of the
chronic diseases of adult life, including
diabetes and heart disease, as well as mental
health problems and proneness to accidents.

FIGURE 3

This figure shows that cardiovascular mortality follows in gradient one's socioeconomic status. Moreover, mortality associated with any of the known risk factors (tobacco consumption, cholesterol, high blood pressure) is less significant than mortality associated with some other unexplained cause.

FIGURE 4

This figure summarizes some of the work of Steve Suomi and his colleagues with Rhesus macaque monkeys. When these animals are stressed, the genetically vulnerable strain respond differently from the resistant strain. The vulnerable brain shows a very high outpouring of the chemical mediators of stress. When these animals are young, if they are poorly parented, they do not quickly return to resting levels when the stressful situation has passed. This shows up as they develop as young animals and is, in part, manifested by their depressed withdrawn state as they develop to mature adults. The males, as they reach maturity, leave their troop and have great difficulty entering a new group. Most of these animals get killed. The females in the vulnerable group that have been poorly nurtured when they are young, will stay in their troop but if they have a child, they will poorly nurture it, keeping the cycle going. If a mature stable female supports the offspring at this stage, the cycle can be broken. The genetically vulnerable males that are well nurtured will, when they leave the troop, tend to be leaders and have successful adult lives.

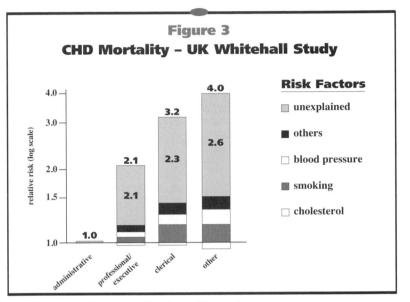

Source: The Canadian Institute for Advanced Research

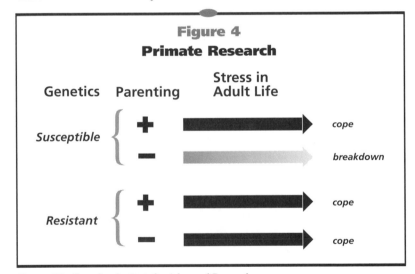

Source: The Canadian Institute for Advanced Research

We now understand how the quality of nurturing in the early period of life sets one's capacity to learn in the education system and to cope with adult life and disease risk. In other words, early childhood development has a strong relationship to the chronic diseases of adult life. We have learned about these pathways from primate studies and state-of-the-art biomedical research, particularly in the areas of immunology, endocrinology and neurology[10] (Figures 4, 5 and 6). The period of birth to six years is critical, because this is when the cortex of the brain is undergoing its most rapid development, which will affect competence and coping skills in later life.[11]

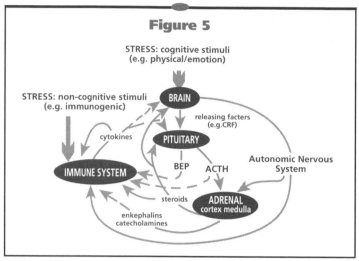

Figure 5

STRESS: cognitive stimuli
(e.g. physical/emotion)

STRESS: non-cognitive stimuli
(e.g. immunogenic)

BRAIN

releasing factors
(e.g.CRF)

cytokines

PITUITARY

IMMUNE SYSTEM

BEP   ACTH

Autonomic Nervous
System

steroids

ADRENAL
cortex medulla

enkephalins
catecholamines

Source: The Canadian Institute for Advanced Research

Figure 6

The Stress-Response and its Consequences

Stress-response	*Stress-related disorder*
Mobilization of energy	→ Myopathy, fatigue, steriod diabetes
Increased cardiovascular tone	→ Stress-induced hypertension
Suppression of digestion	→ Ulceration
Suppression of growth	→ Psychogenic dwarfism
Suppression of reproduction	→ Amenorrhea, impotency, loss of libido
Suppression of immune system	→ Increased disease risk
Sharpening of cognition	→ Neuron death

Source: The Canadian Institute for Advanced Research

FIGURE 6
This figure from the work of Sapolsky shows the body systems that are suppressed by elevated steroid levels.

1.1.3 The Unexplained: Gender Differences

In view of what we know about the determinants of health, questions arise about how these determinants of health influence the lives of Canadian women differently than men. Although it may appear that women are

FIGURE 5
This figure shows some of the relationships among the brain, endocrine pathways and other body systems such as the immune system. A challenge to an individual (stress) will lead to the release of hormone mediators that are involved in the individuals response to stress. These hormones, particularly the steroids, will affect a range of body systems that are not essential to responding to the challenge and enhance others. If the individual readily copes with the stress, the body systems will quickly return to their usual state. However, if the individual copes poorly with the challenge, hormone levels, particularly steroids, will remain elevated depressing body systems that are important for the well–being of the individual over the longer term. One such system is the body's immune system which is an important part of the host defense system. This can make individuals more susceptible to infections. Also, steroids feedback to the brain and persistently high levels are believed to actually cause the loss of neurons, particularly in the hippocampus of the brain. There is some concern that this may influence cognition in behaviour.

healthier than men, because they live longer than men, other health and socioeconomic indicators suggest that this may not be the case. On the one hand, in comparison to men, women in Canada earn significantly less, suffer more chronic and disabling diseases, are more likely to head a lone-parent family and present lower rates of self-esteem. On the other hand, men have more accidents and have a higher prevalence of risk-taking behaviours such as substance abuse, criminal activities and suicide.

How do we account for the large gap in the average life expectancy age between the sexes? Biological factors associated with being female may explain only part of this phenomenon. It has been hypothesized that the importance women give to networking and personal relationships and the multiple social roles in women's lives may have a buffering effect that protects them from negative stress in their lives. But, these and other hypotheses remain speculation at the present time. Our limited understanding of these significant factors in women's lives demands more research, both quantitative and qualitative, on the non-medical determinants of women's health.[12]

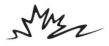

1.2 Second Observation: Beyond Health Care Policies

Our second observation is that, despite our growing knowledge about the numerous determinants of health, we continue to behave as though medical care is the only determining factor of health status. Investments in medical technology and hospitals seem concrete and useful. The public supports these investments and special interest groups (e.g., the health care industry and some professional associations, unions, patients' rights groups)[13] lobby for them. Investing in the creation of an environment that is conducive to good health seems more risky and vague, even elusive. There is limited pressure on governments (or anybody else for that matter) to turn things around.

Our findings clearly establish that governments could do things differently and develop policies that would improve the health status of Canadians. Governments must create intersectoral mechanisms to assess the impact on population health of broad policies in areas such as economics, education, employment, justice and environment. They must develop these policies in partnership with para–governmental organizations (e.g., universities and schools), the private sector and non–profit organizations.

Let's look at how we can pursue meaningful health policies.

1.2.1 Income Distribution

Because health and socioeconomic status are so closely linked, changes in the distribution of income across society have had significant repercussions on health. Between 1984 and 1993, the average income (from all sources, not just earnings) among families with children remained essentially unchanged. Overall, however, the average income of lowest to middle income families has declined while the average income of the top two income groups has increased. So far, income support programs through income tax, unemployment insurance, social assistance and other transfer programs have been able to offset the trend toward inequalities in earnings and limit disparities in after-tax income in Canada. The significance of these transfers is reflected in 1994 statistics: the top 20% of the population earned $22 before taxes and transfers for each $1 earned by the bottom 20%. After taxes and transfers, that gap narrowed to $5 and $1. However, there are signs that the buffering effect of the social safety net will not continue to compensate for growing inequalities in earnings; this may result in a poorer quality of life for the population.[14]

Because health and socioeconomic status are so closely linked, changes in the distribution of income across society have had significant repercussions on health.

1.2.2 Children and Families

Canada spends less than one percent of GDP on family benefits; some European countries such as France, the United Kingdom and Finland spend in the range of two to three percent. Although child poverty rates have remained at roughly the same level in Canada over the past ten years, the numbers are unacceptably high.[15] In 1994, Statistics

Canada estimated that 1.4 million Canadian children under 18 years—one child in every five—lived in families with incomes below Statistics Canada's low income cut-offs, including many whose families had incomes far below this poverty line.[16] It has been estimated that 50% of Aboriginal children, whether living on- or off- reserve, are living in poverty.[17]

In 1994, among lone female-parent families, three children in five were in a low-income household, that is, more than half a million children. Compared to other developed countries, Canada has a very high poverty rate, particularly among lone-parent families. In the mid-eighties, almost half (45%) of lone-parent families in Canada lived under the poverty line (55% in the United States), although several other countries had much lower rates: Germany (25%), the United Kingdom (20%), France (15%) and Sweden (5%).[18] In 1994, the number of non-elderly lone-parent families in Canada living under the poverty line was 51.2%.

We have learned that deprivation during the first years of life can impair brain development and reduce cognitive and language capabilities that cannot be fully regained. There is a clear link between low birth weight and socioeconomic disadvantage; low birth weight is a major risk factor for illness, developmental problems and disability.[19]

The problems of inequality and child poverty are not new to our society, yet the fact that they still exist suggests that we have resisted taking collective responsibility for the health of Canadian children.

The environmental stresses and psychosocial deprivations that accompany poverty can undermine the development of the child and negatively affect competence and health in the long term. Children who are poor have a higher death rate as well as more chronic illness and emotional and behavioural problems,[20] and they do less well intellectually in preschool[21] and school.[22] They are also less likely to develop the cognitive, emotional and social skills needed for success in school. Children from impoverished families have higher rates of injury and their injuries are more severe.[23] These children are also over-represented in the incidence of child abuse, neglect[24] and sexual abuse in Canada.[25]

The problems of inequality and child poverty are not new to our society, yet the fact that they still exist suggests that we have resisted taking collective responsibility for the health of Canadian children. While we firmly believe that the primary responsibility for children lies with parents, it is in our collective interest to ensure the well-being of all children. Child poverty in Canada is a persistent problem, which requires immediate attention and action. Whatever the rhetoric that surrounds the causes and the actual level of poverty, it is clear that we as a Canadian society are not doing enough to provide healthy environments for child development for all of Canada's children. Something must be done. It is not simply a question of money. What is needed is a broad strategy that provides additional money as well as supportive programs that have been proven to work for families with children.

1.2.3 Employment

The impact of economic policies on health status deserves attention. Unemployment, economic insecurity and anxiety, a sense of personal control over one's economic future and economic inequality are interrelated aspects of the economic environment that influence the health status of individuals. Besides giving one the capacity to earn an income, employment serves important functions. Employment provides time structures, the opportunity to share experiences with other people and to link with goals and purposes that transcend one's own, as well as giving one a sense of status and identity. When a household is without employment, dependence on social transfers is unavoidable. This dependence increases the stresses associated with a lower income, a loss of social respect and heightened anxiety about the future.[26]

Unemployment has a far-reaching and extremely damaging impact on health, especially if little or no social support exists. We have found that:

- people who have been unemployed for any significant amount of time tend to die prematurely and have higher rates of suicide and cardiovascular disease;

- spouses of unemployed workers experience increased emotional problems; children, especially teens, whose parents are unemployed are at higher risk of emotional and behavioral problems; and

- recovery of physical and mental health after unemployment is neither immediate nor complete.

At a macro level, no industrialized country has escaped the consequences of globalization and economic restructuring; however, policy responses have varied considerably. On one side of the spectrum, the United States has opted to maintain a high level of employment through fiscal and monetary policies that encourage private investment with minimal government interference. The result is an unemployment rate hovering near 5%, but an increasing polarization of the incomes of the rich and the poor. On the other side of the spectrum, a number of European countries with a social-democratic tradition have established fiscal and monetary policies favouring the growth of high-skill, high-wage jobs, while maintaining a significant government presence to help those in need. The result has been an unemployment rate reaching upwards of 11% and increasing pressures on public budgets, but greater equity in the distribution of income across society. Canada's approach has been somewhere in the middle of this spectrum, always affected by the economic policies of our southern neighbour while trying to remain competitive in the global economy.

We recognize that there is no magic solution to reaching full employment, at least none that is currently known. Some people have recently argued that Canada's high unemployment rate and high public debt have been exacerbated by restrictive monetary policies aimed at keeping inflation low. These people argue that imposed artificially high interest rates stifled economic recovery, increased debt servicing requirements and ultimately placed greater pressure on government programs than would otherwise have been needed. We are not in a position either to support or to discredit this line of reasoning. What we do know, however, is that employment is a powerful predictor of health status. When government decides to change course in matters of macro economic policy, there are always people who pay the cost. From a short–term economic perspective, it may make some sense to sacrifice a few percentage points of unemployment to improve the prospects of economic recovery; however, governments must be conscious of the consequences for health.

The Forum was advised that the main economic policy variable that can positively affect the health of Canadians is a monetary policy that emphasizes jobs and growth.

From both our research and consultations, the Forum heard about the importance of full employment for population health. Current macro-economic policies and excessively high interest charges on the national debt are forcing cuts in the social safety net. The Forum was advised that the main economic policy variable that can positively affect the health of Canadians is a monetary policy that emphasizes jobs and growth.[27]

The Forum recognizes the importance of improving the economic health of the country and dealing with the deficit in the immediate future. However, we also believe that there needs to be a balance maintained between economic and population health priorities. Governments should pave the way for health to be perceived as a societal priority, just as economic development is.

1.2.4 Strengthening Community Action

Despite such problems as high levels of child poverty and unemployment, communities can make a difference.[28] ("Community" encompasses not only a neighbourhood or a village, but also the various places conducive to interpersonal relationships and solidarity, such as schools, workplaces and one's social environment.)

Communities that have implemented various strategies have healthier populations than communities that have remained inactive. Despite the globalization of our economy and major transformations in the labour force, certain communities, regions, and industries have found ways to maintain the dignity of employment for most of their citizens. We have seen that with a little bit of imagination, some financial support and a lot of enthusiasm, communities can act to reduce substance abuse, delinquency, suicide, school drop-out rates, neglect, abuse and violence. They can also support positive health practices such as healthy eating and physical activity; for example, we have learned about many ways that communities promote healthy aging and enable seniors to play a more significant role in society.

1.2.5 The Role of Governments

Non-medical interventions can significantly enhance people's health.

The Forum has collected an impressive list of success stories, which should encourage action

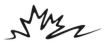

at all levels of government to develop policies and programs that promote health. Medical care is only one way, and not necessarily the most significant one, to regain, maintain and improve health.

Governments are experiencing numerous constraints. They cannot lead in all areas, nor can they divest all responsibilities to the private sector or to communities. They must continue to provide public services. In addition, governments are the ultimate gatekeepers of the common good and are therefore the ideal candidates to encourage partnerships and collaboration. Governments can create the climate and conditions needed for coordinated initiatives to be undertaken by public organizations, the private sector, families, communities and volunteer groups.

In summary, as our recommendations will indicate, governments should act as leaders in:

■ investing in children first, particularly at an early age, and in supporting families (in a broad sense) with children;

■ supporting communities that mobilize to take action;

■ supporting youth in transition to employment and creating "bridge jobs" for older workers; and, finally

■ supporting research on the non–medical determinants of health, because it is a relatively new field of research.

They should also provide Canada, its provinces and territories, and various interested parties with a vehicle to further advocate, monitor and evaluate policies conducive to good health.

All these actions, we believe, must be taken to allow Canadians to continue to enjoy the best thing they have acquired since the Second World War: remarkably strong health. We worry that in these times of hardship, good health will become a thing of the past. Without being unduly alarmist, we believe that governments must act now to avoid the deterioration of the social fabric and hence the health status of the population.

All these actions,

we believe, must

be taken to allow

Canadians to continue

to enjoy the best thing

they have acquired

since the Second World

War: remarkably strong

health.

We have arrived at these conclusions and recommendations from an in-depth analysis of the commissioned work and from listening to Canadians through our consultations. The synthesis of the key findings that support our conclusions and recommendations are presented next.

2. Our Approach

The goal of the Determinants of Health Working Group was to identify the best ways of investing resources to improve the health of the population. At the outset, we recognized the importance of personal health practices and acknowledged that many community interventions support the adoption of positive personal health practices. These efforts must continue. However, while we must take responsibility for the way we eat, exercise, drink or use drugs, for not smoking and for getting the right vaccines and screening tests when needed, these actions alone cannot protect us from the broader environment. We know that these practices are very much influenced by the social and economic environments in which people live and work. Thus, they involve less of an individual choice than was once thought.

The need for a broad approach was confirmed at a symposium on the effectiveness of health promotion held in Toronto in June 1996. The gathering reviewed both Canadian and international evidence on the five strategies for health promotion defined by the *Ottawa Charter for Health Promotion*: building healthy public policy, creating healthy environments, strengthening community action, building personal skills and reorienting health services. The symposium concluded, "It is clear from the research evidence that positive and more substantial outcomes are likely to be achieved if more than one strategy is employed: ... the five strategies ... are synergistic and are most effectively used in combination."[29]

This broad approach defined by the *Ottawa Charter for Health Promotion* is consistent with the approach taken by the Working Group; that is, to examine the factors in the socioeconomic environment that influence personal health practices and outcomes. We consulted specialists for assistance in identifying appropriate actions on the non-medical determinants of health. These specialists were asked to prepare papers on issues of concern for the health of the population related to the macroeconomic environment (i.e., the contexts in which people live, including families, schools, work and communities), as well as on issues of concern for people's health at different life stages. The commissioned papers present conclusions from the literature, examples of success stories or failures and policy implications. The papers present much more detail, and are a valuable source of information.

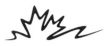

3. Key Findings About the Socioeconomic Context

3.1 Employment and the Economy

The state of the economy has a tremendous impact on health on many levels, including psychological and social well-being. Making a living is a major preoccupation of most adults and produces rewards that affect many aspects of their lives.[30]

Recent economic restructuring has occurred in response to globalization, rapid technological innovation, institutional change and trade agreements. These forces have led to a restructuring of the labour market in terms of both the nature of work and the number of jobs. Downsizing in all kinds of fields seems inevitable. The gap between lower-paid and higher-paid jobs is increasing. In addition, people are experiencing difficulty entering the labour market and are leaving earlier, not always voluntarily. Wage disparities and labour market inequalities are rising, as more workers are working part-time and longer hours and wage stagnation results in widening earnings differentials. There is a concurrent increase in non-standard employment—firms using a core of long-term employees and hiring contingency workers as necessary. In Canada in 1995, only part-time employment, contracting out and self-employment grew.[31]

The sweeping changes brought about by economic restructuring and the resulting transitions that they impose on individuals may have negative health impacts. Inequality in income distribution is a key determinant of population-based variations in life expectancy.[32] One-third of Canadian workers now believe that their jobs are insecure,[33] a belief that in turn affects their sense of achievement, self-esteem, and sense of control over work and life.[34]

There are big differences in the employment situations for youth. Young people (15 to 24 years olds) have experienced an unemployment rate consistently higher and more cyclical — increasing more in economic downturns and falling more in upturns — than the unemployment rate for adults (25 year olds and over). Moreover, youth employment has still not recovered from the recession of the early eighties. The number of 15 to 24 year olds working fell by about 500,000 while adult employment rose by one million between the first quarter of 1989 and the fourth quarter of 1995. What is happening? Lack of seniority appears to be a key factor explaining why the youth unemployment rate has been consistently higher and more cyclical than that for adults. This factor and an atypically weak economic recovery combined to produce the significant decline in youth employment since 1989.[35]

The state of the economy has a tremendous impact on health on many levels, including psychological and social well-being.

Employment and Economy[37]

Canadian Steel Trade and Employment Congress (CSTEC): CSTEC was allocated $20 million by the Department of Employment and Immigration in 1988 to provide adjustment programs for displaced steel workers. The agency formed a committee of business and labour representatives and designed a program for displaced workers that was implemented by teams of CSTEC employees and counsellors. The program services included job search assistance, training, career counselling, relocation assistance, advice on starting a business and job referral. By 1991, CSTEC had assisted 18 projects involving 2,900 workers. Participants had lower (7%) unemployment rates and were more satisfied with the assistance they received than their counterparts in other adjustment programs. Factors in this success included personalized attention, the team's knowledge of the steel industry, active union involvement and flexible, user-friendly approaches to adjustment.

Health Sector Training and Adjustment Program (HSTAP): This organization was established in 1992 to enhance the employment security of health care workers through a variety of adjustment, training and redeployment measures and improved sectoral planning. HSTAP has served 3,500 employees in a sector that may experience 20,000 layoffs over the next three years.

Sweden: Social Adjustment and Health Inequalities: This business–labour–government initiative was designed to reduce inequities in ill health associated with the workplace. The multisectoral approach includes public policy and legislative intervention, research, program delivery and health impact assessments.

The impacts of unemployment vary with duration, cause, and the social context. Socially sanctioned labour force withdrawal (e.g., retirement) is unlikely to have the same negative health implications as the involuntary long-term unemployment of experienced workers.[36]

3.2 Communities, Families, Schools and Workplaces

We are living in a time of transformation. Canadians of all ages have witnessed profound changes in their families and in institutions such as schools and workplaces, not to speak of the information and technology revolutions.

Families are experiencing a time crunch as a result of the changing economic patterns that have led to a common pattern of two working parents. The present phenomenon of children and parents spending less time together has been labelled "family time famine".[38] Families need time together to enhance their members' support and sense of belonging, security, communication and competence. Schools and workplaces must recognize these changes and become more responsive to the realities of the lives of children and parents by creating family-friendly policies; that is, policies that are supportive of the changing demands, dynamics and composition of families. Workplaces need family-friendly policies that take into account the caregiver roles of their employees.

In these times of change and personal adjustment, the quality of the communities to which we belong is of tremendous importance. Our communities are not only our neighbourhoods and villages, but are also the places where people interact and express human solidarity, such as schools, workplaces, places of leisure and so on. We need these "civic" communities for social support and to maintain our mental and physical health in these times of rapid transformation.

3.2.1 Communities that Create Health

Communities are the dynamic groups that people form when they share common space, identities, interests and concerns. People experience community through close family and friendship ties and through relationships where they work, worship, study, volunteer, play and carry out their civic rights and responsibilities.[39]

There is recent evidence that resilience — the ability to bounce back, to recover strengths and spirits quickly — can pertain to communities, as well as individuals. Resilient communities are characterized by the presence of patient and persistent community leaders who have the ability to pull people together, including those who are usually left out, and build cooperative and collaborative approaches.[40] Successful leaders are able to get all players to set aside their differences in ideology and discard such practices as turf protection. These leaders cannot do it alone. They must work with a well-developed and supported network of community development organizations, self-help groups and advocacy groups. The focus is on building trust, finding a shared sense of commitment to community, strengthening social institutions at the community level and strengthening collective commitment to shared goals.

The starting point for building civic communities is not to address problems but rather to identify the assets of the community and build on their strengths. When confronted with adversity, a resilient neighbourhood can pull together and effect desired change: creating jobs, improving safety, reducing crime, ensuring a healthy physical environment, building cooperative housing — in short, doing whatever is needed. This kind of civic cooperation facilitates social reintegration, counters social isolation, helps deal with upheavals in the economy and may even alter the course of governmental or business decisions.[41]

To achieve resilience, a community must foster its own growth and development and value public participation in decision-making while developing and using resources within and outside its limits. These qualities have been the base for the success stories that we have seen. It has been true for communities that mobilized to deal with unemployment, substance abuse or safety.

All levels of government play a key role in helping communities to mobilize. Our changing society brings with it new challenges for governments. They need to continue to fund public services and to create new structures and processes to work in partnership with other sectors. Local governments are under tremendous pressure to respond to increased demands when resources from other levels of government are dwindling and, at the same time, the families and communities they serve are more diverse. *Multicultural communities* require approaches that advocate mutual respect and cross-cultural understanding.

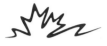

Aboriginal communities can demonstrate remarkable resilience, strength and creativity. Like other communities, they are culturally, geographically and structurally heterogeneous and differ in health status. Economic changes have led to significant social stratification within indigenous groups, and between these groups and the rest of Canada. Aboriginal people and their communities are at particular risk from stresses caused by rapid social and economic changes, such as unemployment. In Canada, Aboriginal communities face poor housing conditions, high unemployment and low incomes. Illnesses such as diabetes occur more frequently among these peoples and their health status indices are worse than the country's average.[43]

As in other communities, patient and persistent leaders are at the forefront of Aboriginal community development. The resurgence of traditional health practices and political, cultural and spiritual rejuvenation should lead to improvements not only in social environments, but also in the resulting health status of this population.[44]

*The **Healthy Cities/Communities** movement now boasts close to 250 Healthy Cities/Communities in Canada, who join over 1000 communities around the world. Successful Healthy Cities/Communities are supported by their local government and are committed to concrete short-term action. They are creative, do not duplicate efforts or structures, are made up of partners from different sectors, support wide citizen participation and show remarkable innovative spirit to develop collaboration, coordination and cooperation. The movement is based on the principle that municipalities are the political level closest to the people and in a very important position to influence their health. The Healthy Cities/Communities movement serves as an instrument for the development of public policies supportive of health and strengthens communities through action across sectoral lines.[42]*

Community Healing

Fishing Lake Métis Settlement: This three-year community initiative focused on reducing high levels of violence. During the three years, 100 of 460 members of the settlement participated in self-esteem enhancement and personal empowerment training. Weekly healing circles were run by trained volunteers. These efforts were funded by the settlement council and the government. The healing circles resulted in a resurgence of spirituality, the closure of local bars, a renewal of community ties and economic development. Many residents are now pursuing education, small business endeavours and addiction-free lifestyles. Role modelling by a core group of residents influenced the health of this community.[45]

Community Resilience

Regroupement pour la relance économique et sociale du Sud-ouest de Montréal (RESO): This local economic development organization focuses on the promotion of community solidarity and business initiatives in an area of Montréal characterized by increasing unemployment, poverty and social isolation. RESO involves local representatives from community groups, business and financial institutions, unions and employers. The program offers assistance to the unemployed, training programs, on-the-job training and support for new industrial developments, businesses and community programs. RESO is funded by federal, provincial and local governments and is trying to become self-sustaining. RESO has helped hundreds of people with information and referral, training and follow-up, local projects, work placement, and workplace training; 192 businesses have used RESO. This initiative stimulated the community, enhanced the hope of the local population and diminished feelings of helplessness.[46] *Its success is attributable to the leadership and capacity of the community to negotiate compromises.*

3.2.2 Families that Create Health

Families provide many of the basic resources people need to be healthy. They educate their members about health, serve as role models and advocate healthy practices. Yet there is a growing diversity among Canada's families, as well as an increase in the complexity of the problems they experience. These elements of diversity and complexity have not yet been recognized in social and economic policies.[47]

The challenge for Canada is tremendous. How can we maintain the health of the population in the face of such familial stress?

First, as everybody knows, "family" no longer means "mom, dad and kids". Increasing divorce rates, a growing number of single-parent families (most often headed by women) and the breakdown of the extended family are all factors that have changed what our society defines as a family. Too many parents, mainly men, abandon their children emotionally and financially when they separate from their partner. Separation or divorce from a spouse or partner should not mean separation from children. Policies must move to a more contemporary definition that reflects the diversity and strengths of today's families.

Second, the problems faced by families are more complex. "Family time famine" is one result of increased workplace responsibilities for both men and women. Women in particular are experiencing stress from extreme time crunches. Women's increased participation in the labour force has not alleviated their extensive involvement in caregiving. The division of labour in two-parent families has remained virtually unchanged over the years, and women continue to spend significantly more time than men on housework and on the care of children and elderly relatives. The double load adds considerable strain to women's lives. Families are also dealing with severe economic problems wrought by the discrepancies among income levels described earlier.

The challenge for Canada is tremendous. How can we maintain the health of the population in the face of such familial stress? How can we reduce the number of teen pregnancies? How can we deal with the increasing number of fathers who have abandoned their families? How can we invest in the development of children when so many are in poverty? Many families have developed strategies to share resources and protect each other. How can we help them? How can we bring *all* families to such resilience, to such renewal in the face of adversity?[48]

Resilience is fundamental to the future health of Canadians. How can we develop policies and business practices that recognize the changes in the structures and functions of families and that help them cope with the pressures they face? With time as a resource in increasingly short supply within families, how can we develop "family-friendly policies"? In fact, the well-being of families should be a filter through which all public policies are examined.

Family Resilience

William Charles Band, Community Health Centre: *Living conditions were poor, housing was crowded, and health problems including skin conditions, respiratory disease and addictions were common. A new health centre created by the Montreal Lake Reserve in 1987 provided school-based immunization, alcohol education, and prenatal care and education. This initiative encouraged families to act as health promoters and providers and supported family relations. It resulted in an increased sense of security about health, public participation, preventive health care and family management of minor illnesses. People who used to live in fear, isolation and despair had a greater sense of belonging.[49]*

Family Matters Program: *This program aimed to expand the informal relationships between parents and others outside the family. The program recognized parents as experts and encouraged parent–child activities and the social exchange of informal resources. The program, conducted in 10 urban neighbourhoods, included a home-visiting component and "cluster groups" that connected families with their neighbourhoods and helped them to socialize and to find common solutions. Child care was provided. The participants compared positively to control families in terms of stressors, support, parent–child relations and activities, and child performance.[50]*

3.2.3 Schools that Create Health

Schools play a critical role in the life of a child. In addition, teachers and other school personnel can have an important buffering effect for children from environments that are less supportive of their development. Schools can make a difference.

School and classroom processes can have a beneficial effect on children who are at risk for poor academic achievement, maladaptive functioning (behavioural, emotional and social) and poor vocational outcomes.[51] Children at risk include those who experience early school problems, school failure, dropping out and difficulties such as conduct disorder and substance abuse.

Programs that target both school and classroom processes, and are under the day-to-day control of the principal and teachers, are promising predictors of school improvement. Examples of successful school interventions include improved teacher–pupil communication, engaging instructional styles and student monitoring and feedback.[52]

School interventions must be sensitive to local needs and the interests of the community. They are more likely to be successful if they ensure ownership through the involvement of all actors in decision making. The interventions must reflect a multidisciplinary approach and be based on a collaborative partnership among students, parents, educators and the community.

Healthy School Environments[53]

Comer Project: The Comer Project aimed to change the school system, focused on prevention, used a participatory approach and recognized the interrelationship between academic outcomes and behavioural, emotional and social functioning. It targeted dysfunctional elements of the school environment. Teachers, parents and health professionals participated in problem identification and solution through a school advisory council, which allocated school resources. Mental health professionals consulted with teachers about students' behaviour problems, academic and athletic events were integrated, and parents participated in school events. The program, conducted in disadvantaged, black New Haven primary schools, positively influenced both cognitive and non-cognitive outcomes of participants in comparison to control groups. Successful interventions like this have low resource needs, harmonize with natural school routines and do not depend on the enthusiasm or expertise of the organizers.

Families and Schools Together (FAST): This prevention program identifies kindergarten children at risk for conduct disorder and offers a full intervention program throughout elementary school. The effectiveness of this kind of targeted approach depends on the successful identification of high-risk children at entry to school.

3.2.4 Workplaces that Create Health

There are at least three primary factors that affect health and well-being in the workplace: control over the work being done, the pressures of work and the support received from colleagues. There is a need to address the work-related determinants of health by reducing the pace of work, implementing more flexible and supportive family policies (including work hours, level of pay, overtime and benefits), enhancing job security and improving social support. In addition, workplace arrangements must acknowledge that balancing work and family is not only a women's issue, but an issue for all society.[54]

Individual worker characteristics, non-work stressors and personal resources are also related to injury and disability rates. At the individual level, the pace and volume of work, the sense of control, the repetitiveness of tasks and the range of skills used are all related to health outcomes.

Organizational factors—such as level and method of remuneration, the quality of benefits, the degree of worker participation in decision-making, the overall management philosophy toward workers and workers' well-being—have all been found to be related to health in the workplace.[55] Greater worker participation is linked to lower alienation and improved mental health, job satisfaction, morale and performance.

Participation and Support in the Workplace

The stories illustrated that organizational change strategies must go beyond those conventionally linked to health outcomes. Changing people's health requires intervention in the social and economic conditions in which people live and work. Organizational change for worker health should involve unions or employee representatives and management. Interventions should start with an assessment of employees' physical and psychosocial health, consider a wide variety of individual, job, organizational and external factors, and address the links among many levels.

Successful interventions targeted interpersonal relations, task requirements and organizational structure; enhanced sense of belonging, job control and mutual support; and encouraged meaningful contributions to a team.

In one project, staff management meetings and career advancement resulted in a 25% reduction in the number of employees with high burnout levels, reduced turnover and improved satisfaction with the work environment. In another project, frequent staff meetings reduced role conflict, ambiguity and emotional strain after six months.[56]

4. Key Findings About Vulnerable Groups

4.1 Children's Health

There is mounting evidence that very early experiences have lifelong influences on brain and body development and the learning of coping abilities. Therefore, the most powerful interventions should be directed at pregnant women, infants, preschoolers and their parents.

During the preschool years, children acquire basic cognitive, language and numeracy competencies that influence later abilities and expertise.[57] Brain development during prenatal and preschool years happens at a very fast rate. Over the first year, the brain matures as connections or synapses form between neurons. These connections create pathways—the brain's map for learning. The brain is vulnerable to early experiences; there are critical periods for the brain development necessary to support some sensory systems.

Evidence suggests that periods of deprivation during the first years of life could mean impaired brain development. The resulting reductions in cognitive and language capabilities cannot be fully recovered. The environment affects not only the number of brain cells and connections, but the way in which they are wired, which in turn shapes competence and coping skills.[58]

The devastating effects of poverty on children have been discussed earlier. Nevertheless, significant numbers of children manage to develop resiliency despite poverty and other disadvantages. This resilience is an outcome of a variety of protective factors in the individual child, family, school and community. These factors include secure attachment, supportive environments and personal characteristics (such as temperament).

The strongest single factor associated with resiliency in early years is social attachment to a primary caregiver.[59]

> In explaining why some children do well in spite of very difficult circumstances, the answer seems to be much the same as that given 20 years ago by psychologist Urie Bronfenbrenner '…. lots of time with an adult who's crazy about him'. Secure bonding in early life fosters internal security and learning through exploration and investigation. Early experience, especially how infants are held, touched, fed, spoken to and gazed at seems to be formative in laying down brain circuits that will govern future feelings and behaviour.
> *John R. Evans, 1996*[60]

There is considerable evidence linking secure attachment to social and academic competence and positive developmental outcomes, such as improved communication, problem-solving, social relationships and grades.[61]

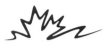

The quality of nurturing and stimulation available to preschool children is a key determinant of healthy child development. Involved and effective parenting, supplemented when required by high-quality child care, can significantly improve children's cognitive and language development, social competence, control over aggression, compliance with instructions and readiness to learn. In addition, the availability and supportiveness of another adult beyond the family is frequently found in children who are resilient despite disadvantages.[62]

To support their children, families need skills and resources such as money, programs and respite (time off). Most families in Canada require non-parental child care arrangements; there is strong evidence that high-quality child care supports healthy development outcomes for children. Preschool experiences foster the development of learning skills and literacy and affect later school learning.[63] Preschools that provide stimulating and supportive alternative environments buffer the effects of disadvantage and prepare children to succeed in school and life.[64]

While the primary responsibility for children lies with parents, it is in the collective interest of society to ensure the well-being of all children. According to the African proverb, it takes a whole village to raise a child—a civic society supports the family and favours the development of competence and of resiliency. In uncivic communities with little social cohesion, more parental involvement and better child management are needed to raise resilient children. Even these may be unable to counteract the overwhelming effects of extreme disadvantage and an uncivic community.[65]

Children

Le Programme Perinatalité (France): This 10-year program was designed to prevent preterm birth. The program employed integrated action on multiple factors and encompassed financial support, education and outreach. High-risk women were visited weekly at home by mid-wives and educated about the importance of reduced physical exertion, increased rest and modified lifestyles. The project was accompanied by a policy of work leave during pregnancy. The nationwide rate of preterm births decreased from 8.2% to 5.6%, work leave rates nearly doubled from 42% to 74%, and the proportion of women who had prenatal care during the first trimester doubled. Socioeconomically disadvantaged mothers and poorly educated mothers were hardest to involve but benefited the most; the risk of preterm birth in disadvantaged groups was reduced.

Prenatal Early Infancy Project: This project focused on first-time parents with risk factors for child abuse (e.g., teen, single, low-income). Home visits by public health nurses during the prenatal period and initial two years of the child's life emphasized education on lifestyle changes and child development, enhancement of social networks and links with services. This focus on psychological, social and economic determinants of health reduced substance abuse, child maltreatment, chronic welfare dependence, child injuries and rates of subsequent pregnancies. The mothers had better home environments; made more use of childbirth classes and other services; were more involved with the baby's father, other members of their social network and their children; used more appropriate forms of punishment and stimulation; and increased their participation in the work-force. The infants did better on standardized developmental tests; were more content; were less likely to be seen in physicians' offices for injury, ingestion or social problems; and had fewer trips to emergency departments.

Staying on Track: This community-wide program in Ontario involved the screening and assessment of children from birth to $5^{1}/_{2}$ years. Public health nurses provided counselling, information on parenting and appropriate intervention or referral, and assessed developmental levels, social relationships and physical health characteristics. The program was characterized by cooperation among service providers. The longer the family was in the program, the greater the improvement in child development, parent–child interaction and parents' sense of competence. The $400 cost per child was compared favourably to potentially exorbitant remedial education, crime control and social assistance costs if no support were provided to at-risk mothers and children.

Hawaii Healthy Start: This program aimed to promote positive parenting, enhance parent–child interaction, improve child health and prevent child abuse. Paraprofessionals screened families according to stress indicators and visited high-risk mothers before they left hospital and with diminishing frequency until the child became five. The visits helped to build a trusting relationship, provide child development information, improve parenting skills, model parent–child interaction, link the family to a primary health care provider and coordinate use of social services. There was no abuse in 99.2% of the high-risk families and no further abuse in families previously known to child protection services.[66]

Perry Preschool Project: This project provided early child care and education for disadvantaged preschool children and education and support for their parents. These children were at risk for school failure due to poverty, minority racial status, limited parental education[67] and stressful home environments.[68] The program included child care and education for children four half-days per week and a weekly home visit by the teacher. The 25-year follow-up demonstrated that the program resulted in a substantial increase in high school graduations, literacy, academic achievement, life skills, home ownership, commitment to partners and children, and good jobs, and a decrease in delinquency, arrests, teenage pregnancies, unemployment and social assistance.[69] A $1 expenditure in preschool programming was estimated to save $7 in later costs for special education, social service, justice and remediation. This program's success was attributed to the children's responsibility to determine personal learning activities and the parents' involvement.[70]

Ryerson Outreach Community Initiative: This outreach project in Toronto aimed to

enhance children's academic, social and emotional well-being by using public schools as the hub of the community and involving the community as a partner in the school. Collaboration of child health, daycare, child welfare and social service agencies led to the development of nutritional, mental health, social support, recreational and out-of-school programs. The program resulted in decreased conduct problems, vandalism and absenteeism, and increased respect of peers, teachers and school property.[71]

Safe Kids/Healthy Neighbourhood (Harlem): This community-based effort promoted safety for an inner-city population in which poverty was prevalent. The aim was to reduce outdoor injuries among children by renovating playgrounds, involving children in safe, supervised activities, offering injury and violence prevention education, and providing bicycle helmets at reasonable cost. Twenty-six organizations, including citizen and voluntary groups, collaborated in this initiative. By the end of the third year, the overall injury rate had decreased by 26%; motor vehicle and assault injuries had decreased significantly.[72]

4.2 Youth Health

Canada's youth need immediate help. Adolescents face difficult transitions and challenges due to accelerated growth, a misfit between school and work, and a change in youth culture.[73] Some groups of youth, for example youth in care, face particular challenges. Many young people are experiencing concerns about the future, diminished self-esteem and difficulties with relationships. Ignoring the changing needs of youth could lead to serious consequences in terms of loss

of human capital, erosion of citizenship and ill health.[74]

The school-to-work transition has changed dramatically in recent decades with economic restructuring and other social changes. Lines between school and employment have become increasingly blurred. High school students often attend school while working at part-time jobs; the number of part-time employed youth has doubled in the last decade.[75]

Job insecurity and inadequate preparation for the job market create pressures on youth. As the labour force skill set is changing rapidly, skill development in problem-solving, communication and social competence is needed. An examination of young people's thoughts on future occupations found that schools encourage the formation of distinct gender identities. We heard that the traditional images of the male breadwinner and female homemaker remain intact despite women's higher grades and substantial educational attainments in recent years.

Ignoring the changing needs of youth could lead to serious consequences in terms of loss of human capital, erosion of citizenship and ill health.

The significant drop in workforce participation for youth between 1989 and 1995 (by about 500,000) has led to significant increases in social assistance costs.[76] Unemployment is particularly acute among Aboriginal youth.[77] Unemployed youth tend to be at greater risk of problems associated with the abuse of alcohol and other drugs.[78]

Recent Canadian research indicates that 18% of young people drop out of high school. It is encouraging that about half of these early leavers re-enter the system and that the number of drop-outs is decreasing. Nonetheless, youth from less advantaged families are more likely to drop out of high school,[79] and within Aboriginal communities, school drop-out rates are two to four times higher than in the general population.[80] Also, the employment gap between high school graduates and drop-outs has widened.[81]

As with children, youth experience increased health-related risks due to poverty and the situations associated with poverty. With adolescents, poverty has been linked to school problems,[82] low self-esteem, substance abuse[83] and vulnerability to suicide.[84] There is a strong relationship between socioeconomic status and educational achievement and career aspirations.[85] Educational attainment is linked to income security, perceived control, skill development and leadership among youth.

Young people are the fastest growing segment of the homeless population; runaways and street youth account for a significant proportion of this group. (Runaways and street youth refers to young people who spend considerable time on the street, who live in marginal or precarious situations and who participate extensively in street lifestyle practices.) Most adolescents leave home because of conflict and physical, sexual and emotional abuse. Youth on the street have different resources and skills to deal with life's challenges. Those who become increasingly entrenched participate in risky behaviours, live in marginal situations and are vulnerable to physical and mental health problems, AIDS, and drug and alcohol abuse.[86]

Tobacco is the most common and hazardous substance used in adolescence. In 1991, an estimated 36,325 deaths in Canada were directly attributable to tobacco use. In 1979, 47% of males and 46% of females aged 15 to 19 were smokers. By 1990, these figures dropped to 21% for both sexes. However in 1991 the downward trend for adolescent females began to reverse, with the proportion of smokers increasing to 26%. Recent survey results indicate that over one-quarter of smokers now aged 15 to 19 began to smoke before the age of 13, and almost 85% began before age 16. People who begin smoking by age 15 double their chances of dying prematurely.[87]

The risk conditions that create vulnerability to suicide must be reduced. Suicide is the second leading cause of death among young people aged 15 to 24, and represents enormous human costs to families, as well as costs to society in terms of lost economic productivity and potential.[88] The rate of suicide for Aboriginal adolescents is almost nine times the national average. Aboriginal adolescents are also at a disadvantage for mental and physical health problems.

Key factors in youth health include a caring family, other supportive people outside the family unit, personal skills and a sense of purpose and meaning.

Youth

The stories about youth projects indicated that group support during periods of transition can have short-term and long-term impacts on youth health. Mentors who offer personalized support to youth promote their competence. Intervention strategies that promote interpersonal relationships, problem-solving and decision-making skills foster resilience in adolescents.[89] High school curricula that focus on life skills enhance prosocial skills and school attendance, and reduce destructive and socially incompetent behaviour. Successful school retention programs build academic and life skills. Primary prevention strategies reach a maximal number of students and teachers, are non-stigmatizing, focus on the school climate, include parent involvement and are cost-effective. Non-judgemental, accessible and culturally relevant support and education services can buffer the negative effects of street life.

Structural and environmental changes also were important. Cooperative work placements at school, school-to-work transition programs, part-time work and volunteer work prepare youth for employment[90]; school-to-work programs involve business–education partnerships.

Community programs can bestow a sense of belonging with peers and adults and teach leadership and organizational skills.[91] Community-level responses to the prevention of substance abuse foster healthy environments that enable youth to make health-promoting choices.

Transition to Working Life for Unemployed Youth: *In this project, a coach met with groups of youth to discuss schooling, lifestyles and employment and to explore job opportunities. Many trainees completed the program and found jobs or returned to school.[92]*

Adopt a School Program (Georgia): *Students with mentors were more likely to enrol in postsecondary education after weekly meetings with volunteers from local businesses.[93]*

School Transition Environment Program (STEP):
This program for high school students of low socioe-conomic status and minority background aimed to maximize the continuity of teachers and peer groups during the first year of secondary school. Youth were assigned to the same class for consistency, and the homeroom teacher was the primary contact for student counselling. Positive outcomes included reductions in absenteeism, academic failures, behaviour problems, drop-out rates, poor health practices, psychosocial difficulties, suicide, depression, substance abuse, delinquency and violence; improvements in social behaviour and achievement scores among students; and lower stress and absenteeism among teachers. Four years later, program students had higher grades and lower rates of absence and drop-out than control students. This successful initiative was low-cost, used existing resources and involved the collaboration of teachers, health professionals and students.[94]

Ontario Youth Apprenticeship Program (OYAP):
This program combines in-school with out-of- school work experience. In-school components include preplacement workshops, skill assessment, job search techniques, goal setting and support. Students are apprenticed in the workplace and given the opportunity to complete a secondary school diploma. The employer is responsible for training, supervising and paying the apprentice. OYAP has been successful because of benefits offered to students, reduced recruiting and training costs, school partnerships with work settings and the commitment of school personnel and parents.[95]

Youth Houses (Quebec): *Troubled adolescents provide opportunities after school and on weekends to learn about other youth and about community life.[96]*

Alexandria Park (Toronto): *An economically disadvantaged community was transformed from a centre for drug trafficking, crime and violence to a cohesive community. The Residents Association strengthened ties with other community organizations and sought assistance from politicians, schools, police and the housing authority. The Association (which involved youth on its Board of Directors and staff)*

offered an economic development project to help youth create small businesses, job readiness training, youth dances and other social events. Community partners provide ongoing support. Young people benefit from practical education, enhanced social support, networking, improved personal health practices and coping skills, job opportunities and career-oriented training. The drug traffickers have dispersed and the physical environment has improved. This initiative, notable for its low cost and community involvement, received the Canadian Centre on Substance Abuse Award of Distinction in 1995.[97]

ASAP–A School-based Anti-violence Program (London, Ontario): *ASAP included staff development, community involvement, student programs, integration of violence awareness in the curriculum, pro-social skill development and promotion of attitudes favouring non-violence. A replication in Saskatchewan had a positive effect on student behaviour and on the teaching and learning climate. ASAP acknowledged relevant issues of equity, power and media violence rather than focusing narrowly on individual skills. Its strategies for transferring control to schools, parents and communities were also notable.[98]*

Youth Services Bureau (Ottawa): *The Bureau created drop-in centres and a range of services such as outreach, housing, counselling, employment referrals, needle exchange programs and liaison between homeless youth and traditional community services. The educational system offered a preventive program for youth at risk of dropping out (a precursor of leaving home), which provided recreational activities designed to improve self-esteem and coping skills. Many youth subsequently maintained school ties and acted as mentors for other youth at risk. Also in Ottawa, the Rideau Centre Youth Project, involved partnerships among street youth, the business community and community agencies. The project helped street youth to gain employment and start their own business by providing space, support, materials and equipment. These multi-agency programs improved the integration and accessibility of services for street youth.[99]*

4.3 Adult Health

It is generally understood that many of the major determinants of health affect men and women differently. However, these differences are poorly understood, primarily because the population health models that are available have been developed using studies based primarily on men. In addition, it is now recognized that women's health depends upon complex interactions among biology, health behaviour and the historical, economic and social contexts of women's lives.

Employment is without doubt, one of the most important determinants of health for both men and women.[100] Employment is inextricably linked with self-esteem and sense of control—important ingredients in mental health. Meaningful work is a determinant of health that should be available to all adults, including those with disabilities.[101]

The current situation of flux in the workplace has an impact on health. Many adults are facing challenging transitions. Even to enter the labour market, adults face difficulties. For example, educational requirements for the work world are higher than ever.[102]

The contraction of the Canadian economy and the accompanying shrinkage of the labour force have significant costs for Canadians in terms of health and health services. Unemployment correlates strongly with a higher mortality rate due to heart disease and suicide. Job loss appears to have more substantial effects on physical health in periods of economic downturn.[103] Unemployment

affects self-identity, self-efficacy and certainty.[104] The unemployed use more health care services, and as the unemployment period lengthens, these people make increasing numbers of visits to hospitals, clinics and doctors.[105] Because work and family are inextricably linked, unemployment can also influence spouses' and children's health. However, the personal resources of the unemployed, socioeconomic characteristics, family interactional patterns, social support and other social factors can ameliorate the effects of job loss on health outcomes.[106]

The average age of retirement in Canada is decreasing—62 for men and 59 for women—and the incidence of involuntary retirement appears to be rising. Many adults have to leave a career job before they are eligible for pension; they have to seek new employment, typically at a lower rate of pay. Retirees returning to paid employment often assume part-time work.[107] Voluntary retirement has positive or neutral effects on health, but early involuntary retirement can have a negative impact on some adults' mental health.

Literacy is an information processing skill that influences access to information, services, employment and economic security. Consequently, reading problems affect health indirectly. Literacy rates are improving in Canada—62% of adults have the necessary range of skills to allow them to read—but rates of limited literacy are higher among people with disabilities, the unemployed and the poor. Literacy problems typically derive from interrelated social factors associated with poverty (such as inadequate educational opportunities, poor housing and disruptions in family life). Despite these difficulties, however, it is important to recognize that many people with limited literacy have remarkable memory, ingenuity and intelligence and are competent workers, parents and neighbours.[108]

There is no doubt that changes in the delivery of health care (such as early discharge from hospital) are having an impact on the lives of patients and their families. These changes are part of the move from institutional, professionally-based care to community-based care and non-professional caregivers. The burden of responsibility now falls on family members. In addition to caring for family members who have been hospitalized, some family caregivers are responsible for dealing with the primary demands of care for members with disabilities,[109] mental illness or age-related dependency. Most frequently, women shoulder the work of caring for family members, despite their increased participation in the labour force.[110]

There is evidence that people who care for relatives may forgo employment, curtail their job involvement by reducing their hours or taking temporary periods of leave, terminate employment, retire early or take extended leaves of absence. All these options can reduce financial security. In addition to the economic cost of caregiving, another effect may be reduced time for continuing education, volunteer work and leisure activities. Despite these challenges, most caregivers do not experience serious emotional illness, because they have resources for resisting stress, such as coping skills, self-esteem and the support of family members and peers.[111] This suggests that there are solutions.

Adults

Michigan JOBS Program: *This preventive intervention assists unemployed people to gain employment and reduces the psychological distress associated with job loss and re-employment. The 20-hour program focuses on motivation and coping and offers a combination of support and skills training in job seeking with enhanced support from family, friends and professionals. Participants achieved higher rates of re-employment than members of the control group; they found jobs sooner and found better paying jobs. Participants also had lower psychological distress. These initial advantages persisted for two and a half years. The higher incomes of participants generated tax revenues that allowed the program to pay for itself in one year.[112]*

Women Immigrants of London (Ontario): *This project provided counselling, support services and employment skills training to immigrants and visible minority women who were economically disadvantaged and socially isolated and who had experienced barriers to employment. The board was comprised of community members. A group assessment of barriers to training, language, technical skills and preparedness for the workplace was followed by development of individual training plans and referral to a training stream. The 20 weeks of training focused on life skills, work skills, language, communication and skills specific to particular workplaces. The program had a 92% success rate in placing its 590 graduates. A key factor in this success was the integration of life and work skill development with job placements and community support.[113]*

Invengarry Learning Centre Intergenerational Literacy Program: *This program provides opportunities for children and adults to learn together, improve their literacy skills and build on strengths. Extensive research was conducted the year before the program was created. Funding was initially provided by the National Literacy Secretariat. Adults attended literacy classes during the day. Early childhood educators provided preschool children with activities to foster their linguistic development. Despite scheduling and logistical difficulties, the evaluation revealed that parents spoke more with their children and were more involved with their children's schools and schoolwork, and the children's linguistic development improved.[114]*

Family Support Clusters: *Family support clusters mobilize support for families who have a relative with developmental and mental health disabilities. Clusters consist of family members, friends and professionals. Staff helped families identify significant support figures and discuss key support issues and strategies with social network members. Long-term changes in families included increased ability to cope with stress, stronger relationships and sense of control, greater understanding of the disabled relative and family context, new skills and enhanced competence in support seeking.[115]*

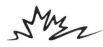

4.4 Seniors' Health

The seniors population in Canada is a large and dynamic group, which contributes as volunteers, caregivers and taxpayers. Most seniors are productive, competent members of society. Canada is currently undergoing a dramatic shift in the make-up of the population; by the year 2025, 18.1% of the population will be elderly.[116] Most seniors are not unusually affected by retirement,[117] although this role change can have a more negative impact if it is accompanied by other losses such as widowhood.[118] However, the average age of retirement in Canada is decreasing, and the incidence of involuntary retirement appears to be rising. This can have a negative impact on mental health through a diminished sense of control, and loss of social contacts.[119]

The seniors population in Canada is a large and dynamic group, which contributes as volunteers, caregivers and taxpayers. Most seniors are productive, competent members of society.

Because Canadians are living longer, healthy aging has become an important issue. Unfortunately, although few older Canadians are destitute, there are pockets of older people—particularly women and minority group members—who are in economic jeopardy. Average incomes for older men and women are highly disparate. Women are less likely than men to have developed the financial resources necessary for a secure retirement, largely because of interrupted career paths.

Limited income due to retirement, loss of occupational role or adjusted standard of living causes distress for some seniors. Income support programs are essential for many seniors. Despite a considerable gain in average income status for Canadian seniors over the last two decades, many remain poor in the 1990s: 19% are below Statistics Canada's low income cutoff. As women have been excluded from many labour force opportunities, many older, single women live in poverty.[120] Forty-five percent of older women living alone fall below the low income cutoff. Poverty is higher among Aboriginal seniors than other seniors.[121] Low-income seniors are less likely to be physically active and to have adequate nutritional intake.[122] There is some indication that poverty is also related to elder abuse and neglect.[123]

When support programs are available, aging can be a healthy and fun stage of life. The well elderly primarily need transportation, money and social support; the frail elderly need additional support because of disability, chronic conditions and medications.

Older people adjust their behaviour to compensate for physical declines. They tend to have a great capacity for coping and for adapting to life stresses, because of their experience in dealing with problems. This adaptation demonstrates their resilience.

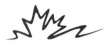

They also adjust their personal health practices. Seniors are active and engage in a variety of activities to promote their health—abstaining from smoking and drinking, eating breakfast, having blood pressure checks and getting regular exercise.[124] The physical and psychological benefits of continued physical activity throughout old age have been documented. Regular exercise can help correct many health problems in late life. Many seniors have one or more chronic conditions that could be improved with better nutrition. The majority of older adults do not fit prevalent stereotypes of inevitable decline.[125]

Older people are, however, more likely to have chronic illness, activity limitations[126] and physical disability.[127] Forty-five percent of Canadians over 65 have a disability; by age 85, 37% of men and 50% of women have some disability related to mobility, agility, hearing, seeing or speaking.[128] Moreover, seniors account for approximately 40% of all prescription drug use, and the prevalence of drug-related illness and injuries is higher in the elderly than in other age groups.[129]

There is a strong relationship between level of education, sense of control over one's life and feelings of contribution. Intellectual stimulation can counter the losses associated with aging and improve learning and memory. Despite physical health limitations, major declines in mental functioning, cognitive impairment and dementia strike only a small proportion (8%) of seniors age 65 and over.[130]

The greatest need among seniors is for services that help them cope with chronic conditions and functional disabilities and enable them to stay in their own homes. The vast majority of care for seniors living in the community is provided by unpaid family and friends.[131]

The social context of the caregiving situation, including social support, can prevent elder abuse and neglect.[132]

The greatest need among seniors is for services that help them cope with chronic conditions and functional disabilities and enable them to stay in their own homes.

Seniors

Days Inn: This hotel chain improved the health and well-being of retirees while benefiting the business. The company recruited workers from senior citizen centres to manage calls for information and reservations. Once the company changed its training programs to accommodate the insecurities of older workers, there was no difference in training times for younger and older workers. Older workers had substantially higher retention rates than younger workers: 87% remained for a full year compared with 30% of younger workers. This improved retention rate reduced training costs and increased the number of experienced workers. The older workers made more reservations successfully (43%) compared with younger workers (38%). Benefits to retirees included supplemented incomes, increased social contacts and enhanced sense of control.[133]

Tenderloin Seniors Organizing Project (TSOP): The TSOP focused on increasing social support, providing health education and facilitating empowerment in a community where social isolation, poor health, suicide, alcoholism and powerlessness were common among elderly residents of low income hotels. The residents recruited 49 local businesses, agencies, bars and restaurants as shelters and lobbied for more patrolling officers. Crime dropped by 18% in the first year and later to 26%. Residents shared concerns about crime, loneliness, powerlessness and rent increases in informal support groups. These weekly group meetings led to a comprehensive nutrition program encompassing food buying clubs, hotel-based mini-markets and a cooperative weekly breakfast program. The residents also opened a health resource centre oriented toward low-income elders and created a tenants' association that decreased rent, improved local transportation and cleaned up the environment. Thus, the seniors became effective agents for change. They felt safer at night and had more social contacts, improved living conditions, better knowledge of safe havens and higher morale and quality of life.[134]

Support Services to Seniors Program: This program, administered by Manitoba Health, provides support services that help frail and at-risk seniors to maintain independent living in the community and to defer or preclude the need for home care or institutionalization. The clients are primarily women who live alone, are widowed and have low incomes and chronic health conditions. Coordinated support services include meals, transportation, escorts, handymen, telephone reassurance and home maintenance. This community program had a positive impact on physical health, mental health, overall functioning, ability to maintain independence, relationships with family and friends, socialization and access to balanced meals. One-third of participants reported that their quality of life improved. The average annual cost per person for this multiservice support program was just $184, compared to nursing home care at $22,000, and home care at $2,100, for a potential annual cost savings of nearly $13 million. The grassroots nature of the initiative and the use of community organizations and volunteers contributed to the program's success.[135]

On-Lok, Peaceful Happy Abode: The goal of this long-term care program was to maintain frail elderly residents who had limited incomes and command of English in their own community. Comprehensive health, social and nutrition services were offered. Support services included in-home care, home-delivered meals, housing assistance, nursing facilities, apartments, day care centres, a respite unit, friendly visiting, delivery of prescriptions, household repairs and telephone support. There were nine replications of the program. A longitudinal study found that participants had fewer days in hospital and nursing homes and received a broader range of less costly community-based services than those receiving traditional institutional care. Health status and functional capacity improved as a result of the program.[136]

5. Lessons Learned

The determinants of health framework challenges researchers, practitioners and policy makers to devise both medical and non-medical interventions that will improve the health of individuals. Current knowledge shows that medical care is only one way—and not necessarily the most significant way—to maintain and improve health.

Medical interventions are generally defined as biomedical, psychiatric and surgical treatments of individuals with identifiable ailments. At any particular time, persons who perceive themselves as unhealthy are a minority (about 10%). Yet there is massive public support for sustaining health care services. People want to protect themselves against suffering, disability and death. Health care insurance probably has greater significance to people than insurance for fire, theft, liability, life and so on. The commanding status of health care activities is due, in part, to the dramatic and well-publicized successes of a number of medical interventions.

Health care insurance is perceived as having tangible benefit; namely, it enables individuals to afford access to prestigious professionals and institutions that can help in time of personal need. These expectations may well be unrealistic and oversold by the health care industry, but the beliefs are powered by hopes, at least as much as by facts and propaganda.

After reviewing the evidence, the Determinants of Health Working Group is convinced that there are key non-medical interventions which offer the public at least as much potential for health improvement as classic health care. As we have seen, some of the basic categories for these interventions include:

- socioeconomic equity;

- employment, especially at entry level (including youth employment) and bridge jobs for adults;

- social support networks (family, volunteer organizations, communities); and

- early child stimulation and support.

These categories of interventions complement health care interventions. For instance, social support services, such as meals-on-wheels, that an individual might need to keep healthy and to spring back to health when sick, are traditionally not part of health care services. Yet, although these interventions do not conflict with medical interventions, they do compete for the same finite resources dedicated to social programs.

The health care industry has an intrinsic financial motivation for providing its services. This financial motivation often leads to an exaggeration of the efficacy of health care services. People and organizations that advocate non-medical interventions, are not usually as financially driven. They may be driven more by moral concerns, political beliefs or ideology—forces that sometimes divert attention from the hard evidence that would support (or contradict) such interventions.

The Forum set out to examine this kind of evidence. We have collected an impressive array of success stories that should encourage concrete action at all levels (families, schools, workplaces, communities, regions, etc.) and by all kinds of players (governments, community leaders, employers, businesses, unions, foundations etc.).

5.1 Lessons Learned from Research on the Determinants of Health

Our analysis has led us to several important conclusions:

- We know much more about what causes ill health than we did 10 years ago.

- We have known for some time that poor personal health practices (such as smoking, unhealthy eating habits or substance abuse) are determinants of ill health, but we now know that such practices are very much influenced by the social and economic environments in which people live and work. In other words, they involve less of an individual choice than we once thought.

- The period from prenatal to age six is critical to brain development. Very early experiences have lifelong influences on brain development and the learning of coping skills. Canadian society has not specifically organized itself to recognize the importance of this fact.

- Family structure and function are undergoing profound changes, making parenting more difficult than in the past, with possible consequences for the development and the future health of children.

- Children who are resilient despite disadvantage frequently have access to and support from other adults beyond the family, such as teachers, early childhood educators and community leaders. Institutions such as child care centres and schools can act as buffers against the deleterious effects of child poverty.

- Economic and social inequities (including poverty) are increasing, along with the accompanying signs of deteriorating health.

- Current high rate of unemployment and growing disparities in incomes in Canada require immediate attention because of their impact on population health. There is an urgent need to focus on entry level employment.

- Because of the transformations in our society and environment, life transitions from family to school, from school to work and from work to retirement are more challenging than ever, with potentially health-damaging stresses for the people involved.

- With rising unemployment, involuntary retirement and labour force restructuring, work patterns have changed, resulting, at least in the short term, in decreased psychological and social well-being.

- We need a better understanding about the social determinants of women's health and stronger efforts to ensure that policies and programs take into account existing and new knowledge about women's health.

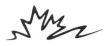

■ Recent trends in the use of tobacco among youth, particularly women, require that legislative and non-legislative approaches be aggressively pursued to protect children and youth.

■ Without being unduly alarmist, we believe we must act now to avoid the encroaching deterioration of the health status of the population.

5.2 Lessons Learned from Success Stories

Just as there is no pill for preventing or curing cancer, there is no single solution nor magic bullet that will solve social and economic problems. A lot can be done, however to prevent massive social change from damaging health. This will require new approaches, new structures and new priorities—in short, a new philosophy wherein population health is a societal goal as important as economic development. We must come to think of investments in strategies for preventing massive social change from damaging health in the same way as we invest in new surgical techniques and chemotherapeutic drugs—not with the hope of eliminating cancer, but as a method of improving the odds of surviving and increasing the quality of life.

The *first lesson* is that, if we want to invest in the future, we must invest in children now. Investing in children means providing money, programs and help to families with children, however those families are structured. This lesson is important because, as we have seen, there is strong and clear evidence that early experiences have lifelong influences on brain and body development and the learning of coping abilities. Failure to invest in the early years increases the later remedial costs to the health, education, social services and justice systems.

All children have the right to quality, supportive environments, including, if need be, home visiting programs and enriched preschool experiences. Access to high-quality and affordable child care or early childhood education should be universal, with parents paying fees on a sliding scale based on their ability to pay.

Society can also help people manage their time through the implementation of what we have called family-friendly policies in institutions such as schools, workplaces, governmental services and shopping malls.

Contrary to other countries, Canada has neglected helping families with children, in particular lone female-parent families. An integrated child benefit program and improved horizontal equity in taxation (from individuals without children to those with children) would help to alleviate this situation.

The *second lesson* is that communities can act to make a difference. There seems to be a winning combination of ingredients in communities that mobilize in the face of adversity to enhance, or at least maintain, the health status of its people. Again, by communities, we not only mean neighbourhoods and villages, but all those settings where human cooperation and solidarity are expressed.

We have strong evidence that when individuals do mobilize to change their community, they can succeed and be rejuvenated if they have patient and persistent leaders, a long-term view, short-term but constantly monitored goals, democratic empowering processes, secure and flexible funding, and finely tuned partnerships and structures. Success is more frequent when the action touches the whole community, with special attention to the people with the greatest needs. Rather than speak of equality of access to programs, these communities strive for equality of outcomes. Community mobilization can occur on several fronts: economic development, employment incentives (e.g., skill building), support to families, self-help, advocacy and so on.

We now know that top-down approaches that lack public participation do not provide the expected results, short-term funding is disastrous, unaccountable or diffuse leadership produces stalemate and stagnation, and neither a single focus nor strategies which deal with many and diffuse issues are effective.

The amazing thing is that, whatever the issue, community mobilization seems to lead to increased security, civicness and resiliency for the community. For individuals, it leads to increased self-esteem, an enhanced sense of control, a greater sense of belonging, improved skills and, ultimately, better health (reduced prevalence of child abuse, violence, injury and substance abuse, and improved mental and physical health). Community action is especially important for Aboriginal communities, for youth, and for seniors.

Aboriginal Communities:
The lessons learned from the success stories in Aboriginal community initiatives are similar to those of other communities. In both types of communities, initiatives reveal the importance of hope, self-esteem, pride, respect for culture and responsibility for community needs. The health needs of Aboriginal peoples are similar to those of other groups and communities in Canadian society who experience helplessness and powerlessness; however, the magnitude of the problems for Aboriginal communities are greater. In addition, given the long history of external control, the impediments for community action are often more significant. It is therefore essential that the external environment become more flexible, accepting and responsive to their needs.

Youth:
For young Canadians, school-to-work and school-to-community partnerships can smooth difficult transitions. Young people can be assisted to develop life skills and interpersonal relationships through student mentoring, apprenticeships and co-op programs. The solutions lie in the community, not solely in the schools. Communities can create decision-making structures that include youth, parents, educators and youth-serving agencies, with the aim of developing after-school youth organizations, community-based employment initiatives, programs to prevent substance abuse and so on.

Seniors:

The seniors population in Canada is a large and dynamic group of people who contribute a great deal to their communities. However, they are at higher risk for a number of problems. A variety of support programs are needed to enable seniors to live and participate in the community for as long as possible. Inter-generational programs and multi-age communities are key to respecting and enhancing the health of seniors.

The *third lesson* is that the most important yet most difficult issue for the health of Canadians is the availability of jobs. We are told that current downsizing and restructuring trends will eventually build a better future. But in the meantime, from a health point of view, it is fundamental that we put in place systems to support people who are facing major challenges because they have problems getting into the work market, they have lost their job or they have left the workforce prematurely. There is an urgent need to focus on employment by supporting people entering the workforce, especially youth. There is also a need to create bridge jobs for older workers who are between work assignments or between work and retirement.

The *fourth lesson* is that knowledge is key to a healthy future. Formidable sums of money are put behind health care services and bio-medical research. However, our knowledge base concerning the social, economic, cultural and gender determinants of health is still thin, and about the efficacy of non-medical interventions is even thinner because such research and dissemination is underfunded. The current trend to rely on private sector funding for research, especially from the pharmaceutical industry, is fundamentally not conducive to encouraging the importance of research on the non-medical determinants of health. We should be moving to balance funding for research on medical and non-medical determinants research as an explicit policy.

In the process of our work, we, and those we consulted, have had to go to great lengths to get access to evidence about non-medical interventions and their success. It is difficult for community groups, researchers, schools, provinces and territories to learn from each other because structures for sharing and monitoring information are underdeveloped. Further, Canada must improve its capacity for information dissemination, advocacy, policy development and health audits.

6. Policy Implications and Recommendations

The question now is, "So what?" What can Canada do to maintain and enhance the health status of its population? We believe that, beyond health care services, a major concerted effort is needed to act on the non-medical determinants of health. Much is happening across the country to create conditions to improve population health, but much more needs to be done.

These times of rapid change and shrinking resources call for action on all fronts by governments, businesses and communities working together to create living and working conditions supportive of health in homes, schools, workplaces and the community at large.

Role of Government:
Our findings clearly establish that governments can do things differently. The Forum has collected an impressive array of evidence, including examples of programs that work, which should encourage government intervention at the federal, provincial, territorial, regional and local levels. In these times, we all know that governments are experiencing numerous constraints and therefore cannot act alone. Nor do we believe that they should act alone even in the best of economies.

Nonetheless, governments are the ultimate gatekeepers of the common good and are therefore the ideal candidates to encourage partnerships and collaboration. Governments can ensure that good health like economic development is treated as a societal priority. Within governments, priority must be given to creating intersectoral policy development and programming and mechanisms, including tools to assess the impact of decisions in broad policy areas (such as economics, education, employment, justice and environment on population health).

Governments cannot lead in all areas, nor can they divest all responsibilities to the private sector and communities. They must continue to fund public services. In addition, they can and should provide leadership and coordinate the various health-enhancing efforts and initiatives undertaken by public organizations, the private sector, families and community or volunteer groups.

The Role of Business:
The private sector, including both small and large businesses, has an important role to play in fostering the health of the population. In addition to providing employment, the private sector has an important leadership role in communities. The Working Group has learned about some important initiatives during the course of its work and is encouraged by these efforts. Family-friendly policies implemented by employers will lead to improvements in the health of the population. Corporate responsibility for the health of Canadians, however, calls for action above and beyond this. It suggests that the private sector can and must move beyond their organizational walls by providing both leadership and money to help build civic communities.

The Role of Communities:

Our research has shown that communities— the dynamic groups that people form when they share common space, identities, interests and concerns—can make a difference. Communities do not become civic because they are rich; they become rich because they are civic. Strong and vibrant communities are characterized by the presence of dynamic local leadership and rely heavily on well developed networks of friends, relatives, neighbours and other associations. Resilient communities mobilize their resources to build on their strengths by harnessing the resources of families, schools, workplaces and other institutions such as hospitals, and centres of sports and leisure.

The Working Group calls on all of these players to implement the following recommendations in four primary areas for action.

■ **Children:** invest in children, especially very young ones, by implementing a broad and integrated strategy of a) programs for pregnant women and for children from birth to age six, including policies supportive of families, and b) income support through an integrated child benefit program and horizontal equity in taxation.

■ **Communities:** invest in local community action.

■ **Employment:** develop employment policies with an eye to supporting people entering the workforce, especially youth, and to creating bridge jobs for older workers.

■ **Research:** invest in the research, monitoring and evaluation of the non-medical determinants of health, including gender, by allocating funds to research on the non-medical determinants of health and striving to achieve balance with research funding for medical research.

6.1 Investing in Children

Canada needs to invest in its children and to view children as a natural resource representing the future of the country. Canada spends less than one percent of GDP on family benefits as compared to several European countries such as France, the United Kingdom and Finland which spend in the range of two to three percent. In the long term, we recommend that Canada increase its investment in children and families by moving toward parity with the mean of European countries. As we have seen, failure to invest in the early years of life increases, later on, the remedial costs to the health, education, social services and justice systems. Spending directed at children and their parents should be viewed as a long-term investment.

Given that family life has changed, families need adequate money and supportive programs to guide their offspring to their full potential. Our recommendations are geared to helping families with children and to creating an environment that nurture child development. We propose a broad and integrated strategy for children and their families consisting of programs and income support.

The Working Group proposes three specific program initiatives for children and their families: home visits, access to high quality child care and family-friendly policies.

Income support is a key element of a pro-family policy which recognizes that the cost of raising children is a shared responsibility of families and society. The Forum calls for improvements and changes to the existing income transfer programs delivered by governments to low-income families with young children. Adjustments are also needed to taxation policies to provide financial support to middle-income earners for the cost of raising children. These two approaches will reduce the gap between higher income and lower income families, address the issue of falling incomes among young families with preschool children, reduce child poverty and provide a bridge between social assistance and income from employment.

6.1.1 Programs for Children and Families

a) Home Visiting Programs

Parents who are identified as high risk may need skills and support. For pregnant women and very young children from birth to 18 months, especially those exposed to higher risks, community-based home visiting programs have proven to prevent many problems and result in better child development and a greater competence for mothers in child rearing and in finding employment. Evidence has shown that successful programs include a focus on nutrition, substance abuse prevention, preparation for labour and delivery, early

childhood development, parenting skills, enhancement of support networks and linkages with other services.

We recommend that a program with regular home visits be a method of choice for at-risk families from the time of pregnancy to 18 months of age. A number of community-based programs already exist and are funded by the federal and provincial governments, through the Community Action Program for Children and the Canada Prenatal Nutrition Program. We recommend that existing programs be supported and strengthened and where programs do not exist, that they be implemented.

b) High-quality Child Care

All children have the right to high-quality care. Most families in Canada need non-parental child care arrangements. Canada's child care system has unacceptable gaps due to problems with quality, availability and affordability. All of these problems create hardship for families and children in most regions of the country. The negative effects of poor quality child care and the positive effects of high quality child care have an impact on children, regardless of social class. Access to affordable, high-quality child care and early childhood education services should be accessible to all, with parents paying fees on a sliding scale based on their ability to pay.

We recommend that governments give priority to ensuring that families have access to such services during early childhood. The different levels of government should work together to negotiate mutually agreeable solutions.

c) Policies that Support Families

Families in Canada are under tremendous stress for several reasons including the increasing demand of caring for family members and friends. This role now goes far beyond the traditional one of caring for children because of the aging population and the reduction of services available in communities. The rate of both parents (from two-parent families) working outside the home has never been so high. Families have never had to deal with so many elderly who lived so long, with so many mentally ill patients who have been de-institutionalized, or with so many people recovering from complicated operations or living with serious chronic illnesses.

Policies that are supportive of families are needed in all sectors of society. Sensitivity to family and caregiver needs should be reflected in family leaves, unpaid leaves, flexible hours, work sharing, day care and elder care. This sensitivity is a responsibility not only of the public sector, but of all employers.

■ Governments and the health sector should play a leadership role by creating employee policies supportive of families and requiring the same of other employers under its jurisdiction. These policies could include but not be limited to flexible hours, work sharing, extended maternity leave, paternity leave, day care or elder care, unpaid leave, caregiving time and family leave. All groups in society should follow the lead of government and create policies supportive of families.

■ Governments should provide incentives for other sectors to establish similar poli-

cies — for example, governments could develop criteria and a certification process for family-friendly workplace policies.

■ Governments should also provide incentives for the private sector to find instruments to support caregiver needs (e.g., reverse mortgages, insurance premiums, advancing life insurance).

6.1.2 Income Support Programs

Canada must address the important problem of children and families living in poverty. It also must recognize the financial load families have in raising children.

a) An Integrated Child Benefit Program

As we have seen, there is an urgent need to address the issue of child poverty. Canadian families are dealing with severe economic problems. The number of two-parent families living in poverty has increased. Almost half of Canada's one-parent families live under the poverty line.

One method, advocated by a number of groups, is an integrated child benefit, which would pay an income-tested benefit to all low income families with children. This benefit would replace the federal child tax benefit and provincial welfare payments on behalf of children with a unified benefit for all low-income families. An additional advantage of this approach is that it would remove the need for low-income parents to rely on the welfare system to provide for their children — they would be able to work and still receive a badly needed income supplement to their earnings.

The federal government could negotiate different arrangements with the provinces and territories to allow for maximum flexibility. The National Forum recognizes that initiatives on this front are important steps in providing an adequate benefit for children. The Forum supports the need to increase the level of benefits for children living in low-income families. A recent proposal of the Caledon Institute has estimated the additional cost to be $2 billion.[137]

b) Taxation Policies that Create Horizontal Equity for Families

A pro-child policy must be based on a consistent recognition of some societal responsibility, along with familial responsibility, for all children.

Canada is unlike all other developed Western countries in that the federal tax system does not take into account the costs of raising children and the reduced ability to pay of families with children, compared to those without. In almost all other countries, there is some form of credit, transfer payment such as a family allowance, or other means to lower the relative burden of all families with children compared to those of equal income without children.[138]

We are proposing that taxes be reduced for taxpayers with children, when compared with those without children. We recommend that the government of Canada institute a process to reform the tax transfer system to reduce the net tax burden (tax net of transfers) at all income levels for families with children compared to those without children. This measure, which would be established to ensure that the net tax burdens fairly reflect families' differing ability to pay, is broadly known as "horizontal equity". Achieving greater horizontal equity for families with children should be an objective of the government of Canada and reflect a commitment to ensuring that every child has the opportunity to realize her or his full potential.

There are a variety of possible instruments for taking the cost of raising children into account in the tax system. For example, a universal family allowance is the instrument used in many European countries.[139] Other mechanisms might include a ceiling on the tax back for the income-related integrated child tax benefit. The mechanism that is least costly and most adapted to the Canadian context should be used, whatever that is. This mechanism would have to be the subject of intergovernmental study and discussion.

Investing in Canada's children also means taking the necessary steps to protect them from key public health hazards. The case of tobacco is particularly important. The long term viability of the tobacco industry in Canada is founded on a strategy of addicting children and youth, even in the face of irrefutable evidence that smoking kills. We also know that second-hand smoke affects children. The Forum energetically supports both legislative and other measures taken recently by the federal government regarding tobacco use.

In summary, The Forum proposes a broad and integrated strategy for children consisting of programs and income support. Programs from the prenatal period until school age should include home visits to help children cope with adversity and to develop parental competencies, access to high quality child care services and family-friendly policies. Income support programs for families with children are needed to ensure that they have adequate resources to meet the basic needs of their children such as adequate food, shelter and clothing. It is urgent to address the issue of poverty among children, especially Aboriginal children. We believe that the components of the strategy should be implemented in the following order of priority:

- *An integrated child benefit program should be introduced to address the urgent problem of child poverty.*

- *Community-based programs with a home visiting component should be supported and strengthened where they exist and implemented where they do not, to help children learn to cope with adversity, and to develop parental competencies. Programs should be directed to those pregnant women and children from birth to 18 months who are at risk, and should give attention to the needs of Aboriginal women and children.*

- *Policies and programs should be reviewed and modified to ensure access to affordable, high quality child care or early childhood education services. Attention should be given to the needs of Aboriginal*

children. In the case of child care programs, we believe that they should be accessible to all, with parents paying fees on a sliding scale based on ability to pay.

- *Policies and programs in the workplace should be developed to support families through measures such as flexible hours, work sharing, extended maternity leave, paternity leave, day care or elder care and unpaid leave. Governments, the health care sector, and the private sector should show leadership in this area.*

- *Taxation policies should be modified to create horizontal equity for families by reducing taxes for those taxpayers with children as compared to families without children, to reflect the cost of raising children.*

6.2 Communities

Communities are vulnerable to the stresses caused by rapid economic and social changes, such as unemployment of their citizens. Community action can occur on many fronts and can have an important impact on health. Our work showed numerous examples of communities working successfully to buffer the impact of social and economic change. Successful community projects were characterized by a high degree of community involvement and support, patient and persistent local leadership, social entrepreneurship, a focus on multiple elements (not single issues), a population-based approach and sustainability.

The goals of governments, the private sector and other partners should be to help communities realize their goals by acting on the non-medical factors that affect health, and to promote community integration, involvement, control and contribution.

Community local development can help people gain more control over their lives and living conditions, thus furthering their health status, especially in a context of profound social change. Such action is particularly important in smoothing transitions for youth and in supporting seniors to live and participate in the community for as long as possible.

We recommend that existing government activities and funding directed to support local community development be reorganized and refocused. Funding of local projects should be based on criteria that include evidence of patient and persistent leadership, coordinated efforts of many sectors, finely-tuned partnerships and structures, focused and targeted goals and objectives with a feedback mechanism in place to monitor progress, and democratic and empowering processes that foster participation in decision making.

Funding could be targeted to support initiatives such as partnership development across sectors. Governments could assist in promoting corporate and community civicness by offering incentives for joint ventures. Some communities and municipalities may benefit from government funding channelled to strengthen local community action associated with the Healthy Cities/Communities projects. In the case where the volunteer sector requires support, funds could be directed to training

and development of a volunteer network. Resources may also be made available to maintain a clearinghouse to ensure access to information about the most effective practices.

But communities cannot do it alone. Partnerships are needed with governments at the federal, provincial, territorial, regional and local levels, the volunteer sector and the private sector.

Message to Governments:
Governments already invest money in community action, although this investment has been reduced in recent years as the public sector has been downsized. We believe that the federal government should better coordinate its activities in support of communities that take action. Frequently in our investigations we heard about the difficulties created by a "stovepipe" approach" to funding, that is, an approach in which each Ministry has its own pet program with little or no intersectoral preoccupation. From the success stories that we have examined, we have identified the need for improved coordination and leadership and for secure and flexible financing.

We have been told repeatedly that the locus of control and management for community action must be at the local and regional level, the provincial and federal levels being too far from the action. We also recognize that, given the diversity of communities and differences in structures and capacities, there is no one model for community action in Canada. The models that we heard about from our research and consultations include the channelling of funds to communities in Quebec through the current regionalization of health and social services, and the mobilization of resources in local communities as part of Healthy Cities/Communities. Our success stories indicate that there are many other approaches. However, in all cases federal and provincial and territorial governments play a critical role by allocating resources and simplifying structures and processes to support local community initiatives.

Coordination across levels of government has been demonstrated by the distribution of dollars through partnership agreements among the federal, provincial and territorial, and regional governments, in cooperation with the voluntary and private sectors. One model that currently exists is the Community Action Program for Children, which is part of the Brighter Futures initiative.

Message to Communities:
Many communities in Canada are organizing to create better places to live, work and play. Whether they are one of the 250 communities that are part of the Healthy Cities/Communities movement or individual communities (such as the William Charles Band on the Montreal, Lake Reserve, Alexandra Park in Toronto, or RESO in Montreal), they have one thing in common: a sense of empowerment to take control of their lives and destiny, and to confront such threats as poverty, unemployment, literacy, suicide, and abuse.

We have seen that many community organizations and foundations, such as Community Foundations of Canada and the Trillium Foundations play key roles in supporting community development. We have learned that these foundations have a tremendous potential for building the capacity of communities to be more self-reliant. These foundations also have a unique ability to create self-sustaining, adaptive local resources. Governments have to find new ways to collaborate with these community organizations. We suggest a new national foundation.

Message to the Private Sector:
There is also an important role for the private sector in supporting local community action, especially companies that make significant profits. As employers, private sector firms can show leadership through the creation of family friendly policies that support employees in dealing with the tremendous stresses brought on by social and economic changes. However, it is no longer sufficient for private sector companies to function in isolation of the communities that support them. As responsible corporate citizens, private sector firms can also contribute significantly to the health of communities and the country.

In summary, intersectoral action is needed by many players—governments, community organizations and the private sector. Coordination is needed from all levels of government to encourage partnerships and collaboration in support of local community action. Governments cannot lead in all areas, nor can it divest all responsibilities to the private sector or to communities; they must continue to provide public services. They can and should provide support for local leadership and coordination of the various health-enhancing efforts and initiatives undertaken by public organizations, the private sector, families and community or volunteer groups.

We recommend that the federal government work in partnership with the private sector and existing foundations, such as Community Foundations of Canada and the Trillium Foundation, to create a national foundation to strengthen community action. The mandate of the foundation would be to reward and recognize community leadership; stimulate the development of required community leadership and share best practices and information including funding of initiatives. Community action should help communities act on the factors that determine health and promote community integration, involvement, control and contribution. Federal money for community action should be used to lever private sector funding. A number of Aboriginal communities have taken action to address their problems. Aboriginal communities may be served better, however by Aboriginal foundations bringing together the growing Aboriginal business community and existing foundations such as the Native Arts Foundation.

6.3 Employment

There is no magic solution to reaching full employment, at least none that is currently known. Some people have recently argued that Canada's high unemployment rate and high public debt have been exacerbated by restrictive monetary policies aimed at keeping inflation low. These people argue that high interest rates stifled economic recovery, increased debt servicing requirements and ultimately placed greater pressure on government programs than would otherwise have been needed. We are not in a position either to support or to discredit this line of reasoning. What we do know, however, is that employment is a

powerful determinant of health status. When the government decides to modify its macroeconomic policies, there are always those who suffer the consequences. From a short-term perspective, it may make some sense to sacrifice a few percentage points of unemployment to improve the prospects of economic recovery; however, governments must recognize the potentially high economic and social costs in the long term, given the significant impact on the health and well-being of those most affected.

The Forum recognizes the importance of improving the economic health of the country and dealing with the deficit in the immediate future. However, we also believe that a balance needs to be maintained between economic and population health priorities.

Although the Working Group feels somewhat limited in making specific recommendations to increase employment, we wish to stress the important relationship between employment and health and the need for immediate remedial action. People are now facing major challenges due to the ever-more-unpredictable transitions in their lives: from school to employment, from one job to another, from employment to retirement. These challenges have health costs.

The Forum wishes to stress the importance of full employment for population health and believes that a goal of maximum employment must remain a priority. In the short term, we believe that there is an urgent need to focus on entry level employment, especially for youth, because of the big difference between the employment situations of youth and adults.

Priority should also be given to creating bridge jobs for young retirees. We believe that workplaces should support gradual and phased retirement through part-time jobs that foster contributions to society. Policies at the corporate level should promote employment through such strategies as job sharing and shorter workweeks. Various policy initiatives can be used to regulate hours of work, including reductions in the standard workweek and increases in unpaid vacations, unpaid sabbaticals, early retirement and job sharing schemes.

In summary, one of the most important yet most challenging issues for the health of Canadians is the availability of jobs. It is fundamental that we put in place systems to support people who are facing major challenges because they have problems getting into the job market or they have lost their job.

This leads us to the following recommendations:

■ *All governments recognize that improving the health of the population depends* **above all** *on achieving the lowest possible unemployment rates.*

■ *Priority be given to helping youth who are trying to enter the workforce, and that barriers that make it difficult for other groups to obtain employment, including people with disabilities, Aboriginal people and members of visible minorities be reduced.*

■ *All government economic policies (both fiscal and monetary) be analyzed explicitly from the perspective of their impact on health.*

■ *The proposed National Population Health Institute which is discussed in detail in the synthesis report of the Evidence-Based Decision Making Working Group report on the impact of economic policies, including the economic and social costs of unemployment, as part of their function of reporting on key public policy issues.*

6.4 Research, Monitoring and Evaluation

The study of the non-medical determinants of health is a relatively new field of interest in which Canada has a been a world leader (witness the Lalonde Report, the Ottawa Charter for Health Promotion and the work of the Canadian Institute for Advanced Research). However, the knowledge base is still limited, in particular about the efficacy of non-medical interventions to promote population health. Further, all countries of the world still lack the type of social indicators ("GNPs of health") needed to monitor social change and to channel political debates.

Canada needs to make monitoring health a priority. In addition, to provide research and policy directions, the federal government should provide Canada, its provinces and territories, and various interested parties with a vehicle to coordinate information and advocate for the development of policies conducive to population health.

With respect to women's health, the Forum supports the recent establishment of the Centres of Excellence for Women's Health that have been given a mandate to develop partnerships and participatory research among community-based women's health groups, service providers, and academic researchers on many aspects of the social determinants of health, health reform policies and gender specific models of care.

We believe that the federal government should make research, monitoring and evaluation of the non-medical determinants of health a priority by:

■ allocating resources for research on the non-medical determinants of health. The Forum believes that the government should be moving to a balance of funding for research on medical and non-medical determinants research as an explicit policy.

■ creating a capacity for information dissemination, advocacy, policy development and health audits. Priority should be given to the following tasks:

■ preparing reports on the health of the nation (e.g., technology assessment, summaries of published documents, analyzed data from Statistics Canada);

■ providing support for research on the non-medical determinants of health, especially for evaluation studies;

■ advocating population health;

■ providing information and infrastructure;

■ bringing research to public attention and communicating evidence about non-medical determinants; and

■ lending support to the development of broader, socially-sensitive indices of human development, in collaboration with international institutions.

The federal government should make research, monitoring and evaluation of non-medical determinants of health a priority by allocating new resources for research on the non-medical determinants of health. As a first step, we recommend that an annual fund of $5 million of new resources be established and administered by Social Science and Humanities Research Council (SSHRC), in collaboration with the National Health Research and Development Program (NHRDP). Priority should be given to supporting gaps in knowledge about the impact of key determinants, such as gender and culture, to supporting outcome-oriented research (especially evaluation studies) and to disseminating results.

7. Conclusion

In recent decades, Canadians have benefited from tremendous improvements in the quality of their lives and their health. But changing times are making life difficult again for large segments of the Canadian public. We fear that the health status of Canadians will soon deteriorate, although Canada invests more in medical care than most countries in the world. We have come to the realization that if we do not value and nurture young children properly, if we do not give them anything meaningful to do when they are ready to work, and if their communities are hostile, unsupportive places to play and work, our legacy of good health may be compromised.

The Determinants of Health Working Group proposes a fresh look at what we know are key non-medical determinants of population health. Although we have learned a lot through our work with the National Forum on Health, we do not pretend to have looked at every important issue nor to have weighed all options. Nonetheless, we hope that our recommendations can be eventually implemented. We believe that the success stories that we have analyzed and from which we have developed our recommendations invite us to begin a long journey on the road to keeping the best thing Canadians have acquired since the Second World War—remarkably good health.

Summary of Recommendations

In order to ensure that Canadians can continue to enjoy a long life and improve their health status, the National Forum on Health recommends the following four priorities:

■ *We propose a broad and integrated strategy for children and their families consisting of both programs and income support. It is urgent to address the issue of poverty among children, especially Aboriginal children. We believe that the components of the strategy should be implemented in the following order of priority:*

1) *An integrated child benefit program should be introduced to address the urgent problem of child poverty.*

2) *Community-based programs with a home visiting component should be supported and strengthened where they exist and implemented where they do not, to help children learn to cope with adversity, and to develop parental competencies. Programs should be directed to pregnant women and children from birth to 18 months who are at risk, and should give attention to the needs of Aboriginal women and children.*

3) *Policies and programs should be reviewed and modified to ensure access to affordable, high quality child care or early childhood education services. Attention should be given to the needs of Aboriginal children. In the case of child care programs, we believe that they should be accessible to all, with parents paying fees on a sliding scale based on ability to pay.*

4) *Policies and programs in the workplace should be developed to support families through measures such as flexible hours, work sharing, extended maternity leave, paternity leave, day care or elder care and unpaid leave. Governments, the health sector, and the private sector should show leadership in this area.*

5) *Taxation policies should be modified to create horizontal equity for families and reflect the cost of raising children by reducing taxes for those taxpayers with children as compared to families without children.*

■ *We recommend that the federal government work in partnership with the private sector and existing foundations, such as Community Foundations of Canada and the Trillium Foundation, to create a national foundation to strengthen community action. The mandate of the foundation would be to reward and recognize community leadership; stimulate the development of required community leadership and share best practices and information including funding of initiatives. Community action should help communities act on the factors that determine health and promote community integration, involvement, control and contribution. Existing federal money for community action should be used to lever private sector funding. A number of Aboriginal communities have taken action to address their problems. Aboriginal communities may be served better by an Aboriginal foundation bringing together the growing Aboriginal business community and existing foundations such as the Native Arts Foundation.*

■ *One of the most important yet most challenging issues for the health of Canadians is the availability of jobs. This leads us to the following recommendations:*

1) *All governments should recognize that improving the health of the population depends **above all** on achieving the lowest possible unemployment rates.*

2) *Priority should be given to helping youth who are trying to enter the workforce, and to reducing barriers that make it difficult for other groups to obtain employment, including people with disabilities, Aboriginal people and members of visible minorities.*

3) *All government economic policies (both fiscal and monetary) should be analyzed explicitly from the perspective of their impact on health.*

4) *The proposed National Population Health Institute, (which is discussed in detail in the synthesis report of the Evidence-Based Decision Making working group), should report on the impact of economic policies including the economic and social costs of unemployment as part of their function of reporting.*

■ *The federal government should make research, monitoring and evaluation of non-medical determinants of health a priority by allocating new resources for research on the non-medical determinants of health. As a first step, we recommend that an annual fund of $5 million of new resources be established and administered by SSHRC, in collaboration with NHRDP. Priority should be given to supporting research in areas where there are gaps in knowledge about the impact of key determinants, such as gender and culture, and to supporting outcome-oriented research (especially evaluation studies) and to disseminating results.*

Endnotes

1. Statistics Canada, Health Division, 1993.

2. Hertzman, C. *Environment and Health in Central and Eastern Europe. A Report of the Environmental Action Programme for Central and Eastern Europe*. World Bank, 1995, and Marmot, M., Smith, G. "Why Are Japanese Living Longer?", *British Medical Journal* (299(23-30, 1989), 1547-52.

3. Federal, Provincial and Territorial Advisory Committee on Population Health, *Report on the Health of Canadians*. Ottawa: Health Canada, 1996, 68-69.

4. Fralick, P. *Youth, Substance Use and the Determinants of Health*. Paper commissioned by the National Forum on Health, Ottawa, 1997 (in press).

5. Statistics Canada. *National Population Health Survey*, 1994-95.

6. Hertzman, C., 1995, and Marmot M., Smith, G., 1989.

7. Canadian Association of Physicians for the Environment. *Brief to the National Forum on Health on Importance of Ecosystem Health as a Determinant of Human Health*, 1996.

8. Evans, R., Barer, M. and Marmor, T. *Why Are Some People Healthy and Others Not? The Determinants of Health of Populations*. New York: Walter de Gruyer Inc., 1994.

9. Wolfson, M., Rowe, G., Gentleman, J., Tomiak, M. "Career Earnings and Death: A Longitudinal Analysis of Older Men", Journal of Gerontology: Social Sciences, 47:4, 1993, S167-179.

10. Sapolsky, R. *Stress, the Aging Brain and the Mechanisms of Neuron Death*. MIT Press, 1992, and Suomi, S. "Adolescent Depression and Depressive Symptoms: Insight from the Longitudinal Studies with Rhesus Monkeys", *Journal of Youth and Adolescence* (20(2) 1991), 273-87.

11. Cynader, M. "Mechanisms of Brain Development", *Daedalus, Journal of the American Academy of Arts and Sciences* (Fall 1994).

12. Kaufert, P. *Gender as a Determinant of Health: A Canadian Perspective*. Paper prepared for the Canada-US Women's Health Forum, August 1996, and National Forum on Health. "An Overview of Women's Health", *Canada Health Action: Building on the Legacy*. Vol. 2, Ottawa, 1997.

13. Commission d'enquête sur les services de santé et les services sociaux du Quebec. Final Report, synthesis chapter titled *Un système en otage* states "The basic problem can be linked to the pressure on the (health) system caused by (interest) groups. The system can no longer assess demands against a more general and fundamental objective of common good, rather than the specific objectives of its various components. Everything evolves around power struggles, professional turfs, scandals and media hype." (p. 428). See also the Report of the British Columbia Royal Commission on Health Care and Costs entitled *Closer to Home*, 1991.

14. Federal, Provincial and Territorial Advisory Committee on Population Health, *Report on the Health of Canadians*, 1996.

15. OECD. "Social Expenditure Statistics of OECD Member Countries", *Labour Market and Social Policy*. Occasional Papers #17, 1996.

16. Canadian Council on Social Development. *The Progress of Canada's Children*, Ottawa: 1996.

17. Royal Commission on Aboriginal Peoples. "Health and Healing", *Gathering Strength*. Vol. 3, Ch. 3, p. 167, 1996.

18. Federal, Provincial and Territorial Advisory Committee on Population Health, *Report on the Health of Canadians*, 1996. The international comparisons are based on calculations using low income measures (LIMs) which differ from low income cut-offs. LIMs represent half the median family income adjusted for family size. (Statistics Canada, personal communication).

19. Steinhauer, P. *Developing Resiliency in Children from Disadvantaged Populations*. Paper commissioned by the National Forum on Health, Ottawa, 1997 (in press).

20. Steinhauer, 1997.

21. Bertrand, J. *Enriching the Preschool Experiences of Children*. Paper commissioned by the National Forum on Health, Ottawa, 1997 (in press).

22. Steinhauer, 1997.

23. Morrongiello, B. *Preventing Unintentional Injuries Among Children*. Paper commissioned by the National Forum on Health, Ottawa, 1997 (in press).

24. Wolfe, D. *Prevention of Child Abuse and Neglect*. Paper commissioned by the National Forum on Health, Ottawa, 1997 (in press).

25. Bagley, C., Thurston, W. *Decreasing Child Sexual Abuse*. Paper commissioned by the National Forum on Health, Ottawa, 1997 (in press).

26. Osberg, L. *Economic Policy Variables and Population Health*. Paper commissioned by the National Forum on Health, Ottawa, 1997 (in press).

27. Osberg, 1997.

28. See the summaries of our commissioned papers which have been published by the Forum under the title *What Determines Health?*

29. Rootman, I. , Goodstadt, M. *Health Promotion and Health Reform in Canada*. A position paper prepared on behalf of the Canadian Consortium for Health Promotion Research, September, 1996.

30. Osberg, 1997.

31. Sullivan, T., Uneke, O., Lavis, J., Hyatt, D., O'Grady, J. *Labour Adjustment Policy and Health: Considerations for a Changing World*. Paper commissioned by the National Forum on Health, Ottawa, 1997 (in press).

32. Osberg, 1997, and Sullivan et al., 1997.

33. Polanyi, M., Eakin, J., Frank, J., Shannon, H., Sullivan, T. *Creating Healthier Work Environments: A Critical Review of the Health Impacts of Workplace Change*. Paper commissioned by the National Forum on Health, Ottawa, 1997 (in press).

34. Osberg, 1997.

35. Human Resources and Development Canada. "Youth Employment: Some Explanations and Future Prospects", *Applied Research Bulletin*, 2:2, 1996.

36. Osberg, 1997.

37. Sullivan et al., 1997.

38. Steinhauer, 1997.

39. Canadian Public Health Association. *Action Statement for Health Promotion in Canada*. Vancouver, July 1996.

40. Zayed, J., Lefebvre, L. *Environmental Health: From Concept to Reality*. Paper commissioned by the National Forum on Health, Ottawa, 1997 (in press).

41. Hamel, P. *Community Solidarity and Local Development: A New Perspective for Socio-political Compromise*. Paper commissioned by the National Forum on Health, Ottawa, 1997 (in press).

42. Dupont, J. *Healthy Communities in Canada*. JMD Health systems Research, Ottawa, 1996 and Hoffman, K. "The Strengthening Community Health Program: Lessons for Community Development" in *Health Promotion in Canada: Provincial, National and International Perspectives* by A. Pederson, M. O'Neill and I. Rootman, Toronto: W.B. Saunders Canada, 1995.

43. Scott, K. *Balance as a Method to Promote Healthy Indigenous Communities*. Paper commissioned by the National Forum on Health, Ottawa, 1997 (in press).

44. Scott, 1997.

45. Scott, 1997.

46. Hamel, 1997.

47. McDaniel, S. *Toward Healthy Families*. Paper commissioned by the National Forum on Health, Ottawa, 1997 (in press).

48. Lord, J., Hutchison, P. *Living with a Disability in Canada: Toward Autonomy and Integration*. Paper commissioned by the National Forum on Health, Ottawa, 1997 (in press).

49. McDaniel, 1997.

50. McDaniel, 1997.

51. Bennett, K., Offord, D. *Schools, Mental Health and Life Quality*. Paper commissioned by the National Forum on Health, Ottawa, 1997 (in press).

52. Bennett and Offord, 1997.

53. Bennett and Offord, 1997.

54. Polanyi et al., 1997.

55. Polanyi et al., 1997.

56. Polanyi et al., 1997.

57. Bertrand, 1997.

58. Bertrand, 1997.

59. Steinhauer, 1997.

60. Evans, R. "Reconstructing the Context for Child Development". Speech presented at the Canadian Child Welfare Conference, Ottawa, November 25, 1996.

61. Bertrand, 1997.

62. Steinhauer, 1997.

63. Bertrand, 1997.

64. Steinhauer, 1997.

65. Steinhauer, 1997.

66. Steinhauer, 1997, Wolfe, 1997 and Bertrand, 1997.

67. Bertrand, 1997 and Steinhauer, 1997.

68. Dyck, R., Mishara, B., White, J. *Suicide in Children, Adolescents and Seniors*. Paper commissioned by the National Forum on Health, Ottawa, 1997 (in press).

69. Steinhauer, 1996 and Dyck et al, 1997.

70. Dyck et al., 1997.

71. Steinhauer, 1997.

72. Morrongiello, 1997.

73. Gottlieb, B. *Strategies To Promote the Optimal Development of Canada's Youth*. Paper commissioned by the National Forum on Health, Ottawa, 1997(a) (in press).

74. Anisef, P. *Making the Transition from School to Employment*. Paper commissioned by the National Forum on Health, Ottawa, 1996 (in press) and Gottlieb, 1997(a).

75. Anisef, 1997.

76. Human Resources and Development Canada, 1996.

77. Anisef, 1997.

78. Fralick, 1997.

79. Anisef, 1997.

80. Gottlieb, 1997(a).

81. Anisef, 1997.

82. Anisef, 1997.

83. Fralick, 1997.

84. Dyck et al, 1997.

85. Anisef, 1997.

86. Caputo, T., Kelly. K. *Improving the Health of Street/Homeless Youth*. Paper commissioned by the National Forum on Health, Ottawa, 1997 (in press).

87. Canadian Council on Smoking and Health. *Fact Sheet on Youth and Tobacco: The Basic Problem*, August, 1995.

88. Dyck et al, 1997.

89. Fralick, 1997.

90. Osberg, 1997.

91. Fralick, 1997.

92. Gottlieb, 1997 (a).

93. Gottlieb, 1997 (a).

94. Bennett and Offord, 1997.

95. Anisef, 1997.

96. Gottlieb, 1997 (a).

97. Fralick, 1997.

98. Sudermann, M, Jaffe, P. *Preventing Violence: School- and Community Based Strategies*. Paper commissioned by the National Forum on Health, Ottawa, 1997 (in press).

99. Caputo, 1997.

100. Sullivan et al., 1997.

101. Lord and Hutchison, 1997.

102. Breen, M. *Promoting Literacy, Improving Health*. Paper commissioned by the National Forum on Health, Ottawa, 1997 (in press).

103. Avison, W. *The Health Consequences of Unemployment*. Paper commissioned by the National Forum on Health, Ottawa, 1997 (in press).

104. Hamel, 1997.

105. Sullivan et al., 1997.

106. Avison, 1997.

107. Marshall, V., Clarke, P. *Facilitating the Transition from Employment to Retirement*. Paper commissioned by the National Forum on Health, Ottawa, 1997 (in press).

108. Breen, 1997.

109. Lord and Hutchison, 1997.

110. Gottlieb, B. *Protecting and Promoting the Well-Being of Family Caregivers*. Paper commissioned by the National Forum on Health, Ottawa, 1997 (b) (in press).

111. Gottlieb, 1997 (b).

112. Avison, 1997.

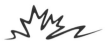

113.   Avison, 1997.

114.   Breen, 1997.

115.   Lord and Hutchison, 1997.

116.   Tamblyn, R., Perrault, R. *Encouraging the Wise Use of Prescription Medication by Older Adults*. Paper commissioned by the National Forum on Health, Ottawa, 1997 (in press).

117.   Lord and Hutchison, 1997 and Marshall and Clarke, 1997.

118.   Dyck et al., 1997.

119.   Marshall and Clarke, 1997.

120.   Chappell, N. *Maintaining and Enhancing Independence and Well-Being in Old Age*. Paper commissioned by the National Forum on Health, Ottawa, 1997 (in press).

121.   Chappell, 1997.

122.   O'Brien Cousins, S. *Promoting Active Living and Healthy Eating Among Older Canadians*. Paper commissioned by the National Forum on Health, Ottawa, 1997 (in press).

123.   Nahmiash, D. *Preventing, Reducing and Stopping the Abuse and Neglect of Older Adults in Canadian Communities*. Paper commissioned by the National Forum on Health, Ottawa, 1997 (in press).

124.   Chappell, 1997.

125.   O'Brien Cousins, 1997.

126.   Chappell, 1997.

127.   Lord and Hutchison, 1997.

128.   O'Brien Cousins, 1997.

129.   Tamblyn and Perrault, 1997.

130.   Chappell, 1997.

131.   Chappell, 1997.

132.   Nahmiash, 1997.

133.   Marshall and Clarke, 1997.

134.   Chappell, 1996 and O'Brien Cousins, 1997.

135.   Chappell, 1997.

136.   Chappell, 1997.

137.   Battle, K., Muszynski, L. *One Way To Fight Child Poverty*. Caledon Institute for Social Policy, February 1995.

138.   Kesselman, J. "The Child Tax Benefit: Simple, Fair, Responsive?" *Canadian Public Policy* (XIX(2), 1993), 109-132.

139.   Phipps, S. "Lessons From Europe: Policy Options to Enhance the Economic Security of Canadian Families", *Family Security in Insecure Times*. Ottawa: Canadian Council on Social Development, 1996, 87-116.

List of Commissioned Papers

Anisef, Paul. "Making the Transition from School to Employment".

Avison, William R. "The Health Consequences of Unemployment".

Bagley, Christopher and Wilfreda E. Thurston. "Decreasing Child Sexual Abuse".

Bennett, Kathryn and David R. Offord. "Schools, Mental Health and Life Quality".

Bertrand, Jane E. "Enriching the Preschool Experiences of Children".

Breen, Mary J. "Promoting Literacy, Improving Health".

Caputo, Tullio and Katherine Kelly. "Improving the Health of Street/ Homeless Youth".

Chappell, Neena L. "Maintaining and Enhancing Independence and Well-being in Old Age".

Dyck, Ronald J., Brian L. Mishara and Jennifer White. "Suicide in Children, Adolescents and Seniors: Key Findings and Policy Implications".

Fralick, Pamela C. "Youth, Substance Abuse and the Determinants of Health".

Godin, Gaston and Francine Michaud. "STD and AIDS Prevention Among Young People".

Gottlieb, Benjamin H. "Protecting and Promoting the Well-being of Family Caregivers".

Gottlieb, Benjamin H. "Strategies to Promote the Optimal Development of Canada's Youth".

Hamel, Pierre. "Community Solidarity and Local Development: A New Perspective for Building Socio-political Compromise".

Lord, John and Peggy Hutchison. "Living with a Disability in Canada: Toward Autonomy and Integration".

McDaniel, Susan A. "Toward Healthy Families".

Marshall, Victor W. and Philippa J. Clarke. "Facilitating the Transition from Employment to Retirement".

Morrongiello, Barbara. A. "Preventing Unintentional Injuries Among Children".

Nahmiash, Daphne. "Preventing, Reducing and Stopping the Abuse and Neglect of Older Adults in Canadian Communities".

O'Brien Cousins, Sandra. "Promoting Active Living and Healthy Eating Among Older Canadians".

Osberg, Lars. "Economic Policy Variables and Population Health".

Polanyi, M., J. Eakin, J. Frank, H. Shannon and T. Sullivan. "Creating Healthier Work Environments: A Critical Review of the Health Impacts of Workplace Change".

Scott, K.A. "Balance as a Method to Promote Healthy Indigenous Communities".

Singer, Peter and Douglas K. Martin. "Improving Dying in Canada".

Steinhauer, Paul D. "Developing Resiliency in Children from Disadvantaged Populations".

Sudermann, Marlies and Peter G. Jaffe. "Preventing Violence: School- and Community-Based Strategies".

Sullivan, T. , O. Uneke, J. Lavis, D. Hyatt and J. O'Grady. "Labour Adjustment Policy and Health: Considerations for a Changing World".

Tamblyn, Robyn and Robert Perreault. "Encouraging the Wise Use of Prescription Medication by Older Adults".

Wolfe, David A. "Prevention of Child Abuse and Neglect".

Zayed, Joseph and Luc Lefebvre. "Environmental Health: From Concept to Reality".

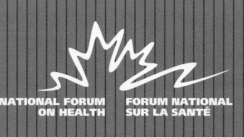

NATIONAL FORUM ON HEALTH   **FORUM NATIONAL SUR LA SANTÉ**

Creating a Culture of Evidence-Based Decision Making in Health

Evidence-Based Decision Making Working Group

Karen Gainer, LL.B. (Chair)
Mamoru Watanabe, M.D. (Chair)
Rober G. Evans, Ph.D.
Margaret McDonald, R.N.
Eric M. Maldoff, LL.B.
Tom W. Noseworthy, M.D.
Noralou P. Roos, Ph.D.
Lynn Smith, LL.B., Q.C.

Kayla Estrin (Policy Analyst)
Krista Locke (Policy Analyst)

Contents

Introduction 3

Making Decisions 4

Accountability 5

Evidence-Based Decision Making 6

The Vision of an Evidence-Based Health System 7

Why Do We Need Evidence-Based Decision Making Now? 8

    Population health and determinants of health 8

    Controlling health care costs: effectiveness and efficiency 8

    Health information and health care reform 9

    Research and emerging issues 10

    Needs of patients and users 10

Barriers to Use of Evidence 12

    Lack of useful evidence 12

    Lack of consensus 13

    Inappropriate use of evidence 13

    Lag time in diffusion and uptake of information 14

    Overwhelming amounts of information 14

    Decisions made without consideration of health outcomes 15

    Differing and changing values 16

    Lack of accountability 16

    Tradition and judgment 17

    Privacy and confidentiality of information 17

    Uncoordinated development of health information systems 19

How Do We Know That We Need to Improve the Use of Evidence? 20

Signs of Progress 21

Achieving the Vision 24

Leadership 26

Improving Public Accountability Through a Nation-Wide Health Information System 26

Research and Evaluation 29

Funding 31

Improving Dissemination and Uptake of Evidence 32

Balancing Privacy and Accessibility of Health Information 34

Conclusion 35

References 37

Appendix 1 41

Introduction

The National Forum on Health believes that one of the key goals of the health sector in the 21st century should be the establishment of a culture of evidence-based decision making. Decision makers at all levels—health care providers, administrators, policy makers, patients and the public—will use high-quality evidence to make informed choices about health and health care.

The Evidence-Based Decision Making Working Group investigated and debated possible strategies that would insert more high-quality evidence into the decision-making process at the level of both practice and policy; that would make decision making more accountable; and that would produce the best possible health and health care outcomes.

The Working Group commissioned research to:

■ examine the meaning and concepts of evidence and evidence-based decision making;

■ identify cases of successful implementation of evidence-based decision making as well as cases that illustrate opportunities for improvement;

■ identify the health information infrastructure needed to support evidence-based decision making;

■ examine tools which support more effective health care decision making; and

■ identify strategies for assisting and increasing the role of Canadians in decision making in health and health care.

We heard from the public and key stakeholders through public consultations, national stakeholder conferences and dialogues with consumers and experts of health information technology (see Appendix 1).

This paper summarizes our findings. It begins with a brief description of evidence-based decision making and the barriers to the use of evidence, explaining why these problems exist and describing some of the factors which influence the use of evidence. We then present our vision of an evidence-based culture for health and health care and the means to create this culture. The final section offers opportunities and solutions to achieve this vision.

Making Decisions

Decisions about health and health care are made daily at all levels — at the level of policy and regulation, management and administration, and in individual health care, as illustrated by the following scenarios. Some decisions have good outcomes, others have unfortunate consequences which might have been avoided with better information.

The Board of a large metropolitan hospital is required to decide how best to manage a $1.2 million budget cut. The chair searches for supportive evidence to help the Board formulate a rational response. He asks for performance indicators on how the hospital compares with others to determine potential cost-saving strategies and optimal budget allocations which would not sacrifice patient and provider needs. He is told that, although large amounts of data are available, the information is not useful for making budgetary decisions and, at the end of the day, program trade-offs are made with little evidence to support the final decisions.

Health and health care decisions are complex and tough. While some decisions are grounded on sound evidence, many are not. Evidence is but one of the elements in decision making. The values and interests of the decision maker, as well as the situation or context in which the decision is being made, influence the process and outcome.

Applying the best available evidence in the decision-making process does not in itself guarantee good decisions or outcomes, but it does improve the odds of both. We believe that using the best available evidence is key to improving decisions and outcomes that affect health.

A 40-year-old female executive of a major national organization visits her family physician for an annual physical examination. Although she is feeling well, she reveals that her 65- year-old mother died recently of colorectal cancer, making her the second generation to succumb to this disease. The physician and the patient, both concerned with the family history, want to find current information about the risks and prognosis and what potential preventive strategies might be available. Unable to find information specific to her ethnic origins, lifestyle and socioeconomic status, the family physician refers her to the Cancer Society for the information. While a great deal of high-quality evidence is available from that source, she does not believe it is relevant to her.

Accountability

A provincial government looking for ways to solve the problems of growing health inequities across geographic regions and sub-populations, and increasing health care costs, convenes a task force to advise on how to get the most out of its health care expenditures and to address the health inequities. In its consultations, the task force is told consistently that communities, regions and individuals must have a greater voice in making decisions about health and health care. The government acts on this advice by decentralizing its authority and transferring its control to regional authorities. Having made this decision with little supporting evidence that regionalization will address the problem, the government is faced with evaluating the effectiveness and efficiency of this decision when real costs do not decrease as expected, and health inequities remain.

Demonstrating that health services have been effective and efficient is not a simple task. There are varying degrees of evidence on which current practice and policy decisions are based. Many decisions about management and funding of health services are based on nothing at all or fragmentary pieces of evidence, stitched together with a good measure of judgment.

The ultimate goals for everything we do in the health system are to improve health status and quality of life. Ideally, those who provide services and manage the health system should be able to demonstrate that services and programs have improved health beyond that which would have been achieved by doing something else with the same resources, or by doing nothing at all. (Brtitish Columbia Provincial Health Officer, 1996)

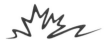

Evidence-Based Decision Making

> *It is incredible what we don't know; but incredible the amount of information we have and don't use. As a result costly health and health care decisions are made based on little or no evidence.*
>
> Robert G. Evans,
> Health Economist

How can we foster a culture of evidence-based decision making throughout a health care system where, on the one hand much information is lacking about many questions, and on the other hand there exists an overwhelming amount of information that is not used? As a first step in analyzing this question, we need to understand what evidence-based decision making is and is not.

Evidence-based decision making is the systematic application of the best available evidence to the evaluation of options and to decision making in clinical, management and policy settings.

Evidence-based medicine has received increasing attention over the last decade, as priority has been given to bringing the best available clinical evidence to the attention of practitioners, particularly physicians. But individuals, administrators and policy makers equally need the best available evidence on which to base their decisions regarding health and health care.

Best available evidence can be obtained from diverse and extensive sources. Multi-disciplinary research brings methodologies and results from different disciplines with different limitations. Although randomized clinical trials, described as the "gold standard" of evidence, are important sources of information, they too have limitations. Other methodologies can also contribute sound and important sources of information. The key is for the decision maker to understand the limitations of the evidence at hand, and the impact and relevance it will have on decision outcomes.

It is also helpful to understand what evidence-based decision making is not. It is not tyranny over providers; it is not value free; it is not a suggestion that evidence is not being used now; it is not a methodological strait-jacket; and it is not an excuse for inaction. Nor is evidence-based decision making based solely on evidence. It is influenced by individual values, interests and judgments as well as external pressures and conditions. It is simply getting the best information in place so that people can make the best decision which is consistent with their values and circumstances.

We believe that evidence-based decision making should be the foundation for an effective and efficient health system.

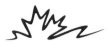

Waiting for perfect evidence is no excuse for ignoring available information or for doing nothing. Health and health care are dynamic processes; research within and outside the health system influences health and health care issues every day. Evidence is continually changing. The culture must continually adapt and progress until the use of best available evidence is explicit and carries a greater weight in decision making.

The Vision of an Evidence-Based Health System

In an evidence-based health system, sufficient, useful evidence is available for all health and health care decisions. Information systems and technology are state of the art. Decision makers at all levels of the health system are able to get access to relevant and timely information on population health strategies and both medical and non-medical health determinants. Information is integrated and readily accessible from all health sectors and from other sectors which affect health.

Incentives and tools are in place to ensure that the best evidence is used. Decision making is accountable and transparent. An efficient and effective health system exists which contributes to improved health status and quality of life.

■ Patients have access to best-quality, easy-to-assimilate information on their health status and treatment choices which are appropriate to their gender and other personal characteristics. Risks and benefits for each treatment are fully explained to the patient by the health care team. Additional information is readily available through easy-to-use, automated and non-automated patient support tools in a language that is understood. The informed patient is involved in choice of treatment. Only appropriate interventions are employed, and patient education is gender and culturally specific.

■ Administrators of health care services and institutions including home care, mental health and community health have access to longitudinal and comparative data on service variations. Short- and long-term performance indicators exist. Integrated, linked information on socioeconomic indicators, medical and non-medical determinants of health, utilization costs and health care capacity are available. Information systems provide comparative analyses across planning areas, leading to the understanding of the relative contributions of non-medical and medical inputs to health; the linkage of information to current funding and delivery perspectives; and the flexibility to provide focused responses to well-articulated policy questions.

■ Providers have access to high-quality patient care evidence at the point of care. The evidence is as specific to the situation as possible taking all relevant differences, including gender and culture, into consideration. Information on standards of practice and cost evaluations are readily available. High-quality evidence, with appropriate incentives and tools, enables adoption of new approved standards of practice. Health and medical records distributed over a number of institutions and organizations are accessible as needed through information technology which guarantees privacy and confidentiality of patient records.

■ Policy makers have access to patient care and cost benefit information in aggregate form to protect patient privacy, and information on the priorities, interests and values of their constituents. Longitudinal studies and projections are readily available, and an effective forum for stakeholder debate and involvement exists.

Why Do We Need Evidence-Based Decision Making Now?

A number of factors and emerging trends that have an impact on the health care system are placing more emphasis on the need for evidence in making decisions. A growing focus on population health and its determinants, greater fiscal pressures, new information and knowledge created by research and advances in technology, and the health and health care reform movement are demanding better decision making.

Population health and determinants of health

We know now, better than we did before, what makes people healthy. We know, for example, that employment and income (often tied to education), are critical to maintaining our sense of dignity, the health of our bodies and minds, and our immune system's ability to ward off infection and disease. While our knowledge about health determinants is improving, we need further analysis to assist us in incorporating this new knowledge in making decisions about health and health care at the individual level.

Controlling health care costs: effectiveness and efficiency

The move towards evidence-based decision making is also being driven by fiscal restraint. Health care costs have risen disproportionately to the marginal improvement in health status. From 1975 to 1993, real per capita health expenditures increased from approximately $1,100 to $2,000 (Health Canada, 1996). We know that spending more money on health care does not necessarily lead to better health. The quest to balance budgets and reduce indebtedness at all levels of government has accelerated the speed of change in the health sector. Accordingly, with greater fiscal pressures on our health care budget, we must use best evidence to help us allocate finite resources to improve health care services and health status. This is fundamental to improving efficiency and effectiveness.

Like other health care decision makers, administrators and policy makers need evidence on the medical and non-medical determinants of health, and on the effectiveness of interventions. But they also need to know the relative costs of available alternatives.

Data that allow for comparison of program and service costs with other models of delivery and assessment of the cost of practice variations are far from available. Although some data bases do exist which are rich with various types of data, many are not integrated or linked to enable comparisons of intermediate and long-term service performance. Ideally, service cost and socio-demographic and clinical determinants data have to be linked and available at the individual patient level.

At the macro level, decisions about hospital closures, primary care restructuring and policies on continuing care services, to name a few, are under way, and decision makers are finding that the facts and figures they need are unavailable.

Health information and health care reform

Advances in information systems and information and networking technologies enable decision makers to get information and relevant evidence more efficiently than ever before. Although management information systems in the health sector are lagging far behind other sectors such as banking, there are promising signs that such systems can assist evidence-based decision making at all levels of our health system.

We know that spending more money on health care does not necessarily lead to better health.

As health information systems advance, more accessible, complex and comprehensive data provide impressive opportunities to improve decision making. However, such a wealth of data correspondingly calls for a much greater capacity to produce integrated and linked information at the individual patient level. Technological innovations have created the capacity for integrating and linking data bases while protecting privacy and confidentiality. Many studies of health reform in Canada have stated that this would not be possible without the effective use of information technology (CANARIE, 1996).

Regionalization and decentralization of our health care system require effective monitoring of performance standards and accurate information on how health care resources are being utilized, providing a method to compare with other regions. Data on health outcomes provide the opportunity to judge the effectiveness of existing and new health interventions.

Decentralization and regionalization will place more demands on administrators for accountability about decisions and their health outcomes. They will need to report on the health status of the region and improve the public's understanding of the relationship between medical and non-medical determinants of health and the burden of disease. Concurrently, the regional body will receive assurance that the best possible services are being provided and that wasteful practices are being minimized. Information systems and technology have the potential to make great strides toward increasing accountability of decision makers and improving decision making.

Research and emerging issues

Although advances in research are contributing to a broader information base, they are demanding better approaches to evaluating this information, incorporating the new with existing knowledge. What may appear to be conflicting or ambiguous data require thoughtful interpretation. In response, many health care providers, policy makers and administrators are looking for critical analysis, systematic reviews and synthesis of available evidence which distill knowledge to enable best practice and optimal policy decisions.

New information which is dependent on effective scanning of the environment also arises through natural experiments. For example, the geographical distribution of physicians' work raises the question, "Does a jurisdiction functioning with many more physicians per capita than another provide health advantages to the population?"

New issues are continually forcing decision makers to confront the question of whether policy decisions and their interventions are appropriate. For example, the increasing incidence of peanut oil sensitivity is causing some school cafeterias and airlines to consider eliminating peanut products from their menus. Society may soon have to determine whether and when such sensitivities will demand that peanuts be declared a product potentially hazardous to health, as in the case of tobacco. Without systematic collection of data and appropriate information, how and when will we decide that something becomes a public health issue with significant health care implications requiring intervention?

Needs of patients and users

The increasing amount of information and improvements in communication strategies are encouraging, and are enabling patients and the public at large to become more informed. Patients are asking for more information on disease and treatment options, and the public has told us that they wish to become more influential in health policy and program issues. They express an increasing reluctance to leaving system-wide decisions in the hands of experts and governments. While some professionals may believe that the public exert little influence on policy and practice issues, some examples suggest otherwise. For instance, the public have played a significant role in supporting development of acupuncture programs in some provinces; and in the development and implementation of culturally sensitive addictions programs in First Nations and Inuit communities. And survivors of breast cancer have also had significant impact on health care policy. As a result of advocacy, survivors are working on committees of the Canadian Breast Cancer Initiative to provide advice on setting the research agenda, and on developing clinical guidelines for cure and treatment of patients with breast cancer.

We are all aware that rumours and inaccurate information can sabotage uptake of best available evidence. Accordingly, there is an urgent need for the dissemination of more accurate information to challenge the myths and misinformation surrounding our health system. Improved access to relevant and accurate information about health status and treatment options will help to address the problem of decisions being made using inappropriate and poor-quality evidence.

We have an admirable history of organizations lobbying for changes to the health system. Less developed is activism on the part of the individual in his/her personal treatment regimen. In the United States, a magazine aimed at health care consumers, called *Health Pages*, offers rating guides to local physicians, hospitals and insurance plans, along with more generic articles on health. Similarly, a best-selling home medical guide called *Take Care of Yourself* (Vickey and Fries, 1992) helps consumers determine if, when or how quickly they need to visit the doctor when they experience a wide range of symptoms. There are also a number of Canadian books available on a variety of health topics.

In Canada the first *Report on the Health of Canadians* released in 1996 details a variety of national health indicators, describes the prevalence of various illnesses and points at

the determinants of health and well-being by comparing health status to income level and level of education (F/P/T Advisory Committee on Population Health, 1996). The Report helps to measure Canada's progress in achieving better overall health of the population. We endorse this initiative but acknowledge that more information is needed which assists the public to become more involved in making decisions about their own health and influencing health policy in Canada. The Report does not help us understand how health is (or is not) related to the relative utilization of health care.

The Forum believes that population health, health services and health system data currently available are scant in comparison to what would be required if we were to reduce the asymmetry of information between health policy makers, administrators and health care providers on the one hand and users of services on the other. Information should be widely available in a format that educates and informs the public and provides an incentive to be more active in the administration of care.

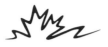

Barriers to Use of Evidence

While many debate the outcomes and consequences of these activities and trends, the benefit of evidence-based decision making is well recognized. Work is already under way to remove barriers to using best evidence. Much more work is required.

To have a more effective and efficient health system, evidence-based decision making must be universally and consistently adopted by providers, administrators, policy makers, patients and the public at large. However, we have noted that problems and barriers to using good evidence exist for all decision makers.

For some decisions, high-quality evidence simply does not exist or is not useful because it is not relevant, accessible or timely enough for operational needs. For other decisions, the evidence used is inappropriate or of poor quality. Some decisions are made without recourse to useful and relevant information available. In some instances, decisions are made on evidence directed toward a non-health outcome but which has an impact on health or health care.

Lack of useful evidence

On the one hand, research is generating volumes of new evidence. On the other hand, in numerous instances evidence is still not available, is insufficient to support practices and treatments, or is not useful because it is not understood. Given the pace of new knowledge generation, the available evidence in accessible format may be quickly outdated, with the new knowledge yet to be synthesized and translated.

Information that is available is often not useful. More user-friendly interfaces must be developed so that decision makers know how to find and use the information to make better decisions. Further, information must be available in a language that is understood by the user. Critical analyses, systematic reviews and translation of the available information will help address these problems.

In the clinical realm, much of the promotion of many alternative, or non-conventional, medicines and therapies is based either on insufficient, poor-quality or inappropriate evidence. Statistics Canada numbers show that over three million Canadians spent $1 billion last year for alternative treatments not covered by traditional health plans (Walters, 1996). As a result of growing public interest in alternative treatments, conventional institutions are starting to raise questions about the appropriate place of alternative interventions such as acupuncture, herbology and chiropractics.

During our public consultations, we heard support for alternative and complementary therapies provided that their effectiveness is demonstrated. We believe that these therapies should be assessed using appropriate methods, which are intended to reduce bias, to determine the effect on health status outcomes. This need for assessment also applies to a wide array of therapies that are currently used in conventional clinical practice.

Although there is a reasonable understanding of clinical outcomes at the level of individual health, we need to help patients, clinicians and the public understand the relative importance of clinical interventions (e.g., drugs, surgery) versus non-clinical interventions (e.g., investments in early childhood education, job enrichment, job retraining). While we have good evidence on the effectiveness of both types of efforts, we know little about their relative cost effectiveness in improving health. There is insufficient information on how to translate determinants of health concepts into an implementation strategy to improve population health status. Synthesis and translation of existing knowledge about non-medical determinants are critical for better decision making.

Lack of consensus

Even when there is information about the outcomes of some clinical practices and treatments, providers may sometimes find it difficult to understand, perhaps reflective of conflicting expert opinions or information which is ambiguous, inconclusive or not relevant or specific enough to the practice or policy at hand. For example, although cholesterol screening is widely used and practice guidelines have been developed, some argue that there is insufficient evidence to support this practice. While experts agree that lowering blood cholesterol levels may reduce the incidence of ischemic heart disease in men between the ages of 30 and 59, they question the long-term safety and efficacy of cholesterol-lowering drugs and their impact on the overall death rate (Canadian Task Force on the Periodic Health Examination, 1994). As a result, current practice varies considerably in this area.

Evidence can vary in the degree to which it is a persuasive force for different decision makers. What is compelling evidence for one decision maker may be considered insufficient or of poor quality by another. This fact emphasizes the role of interests, values, experience, judgment and other factors in the decision-making process.

Inappropriate use of evidence

Applying the findings of many research studies to populations which include all gender, race and age groups is an example of the inappropriate use of evidence. Much research is done only on adult males, making it difficult to know if the interventions, including pharmaceutical treatments, are applicable to the Canadian population at large, and if these interventions are indeed safe and effective when applied to groups that have not been included in the study.

A recent assessment of randomized clinical trials for gender and cultural bias has indicated that in certain areas, women and people in disadvantaged groups have been underrepresented in clinical trials (Judelson, 1995; Kitler, 1994). Genetic, behavioural and psychosocial differences as well as hormonal status potentiate differences in the responsiveness of specific population groups to medical interventions (LaRosa and Alexander, 1995). It is unsound

Evidence can vary in the degree to which it is a persuasive force for different decision makers.

practice to administer a drug or other intervention to a group on which the intervention has not been tested. Research should benefit all people, and populations should not be treated with interventions that have not been tested on them. Legal restrictions designed to protect population groups from research risk may actually expose them to greater risk.

Misinformation which exists in the health system often leads to poor choices. Although there is evidence that generic drugs are as good as higher cost brand name drugs, patients continue to ask for the brand name drugs, because of inaccurate perceptions that generic drugs are made with cheaper and, therefore, less effective or more harmful ingredients.

Strongly held beliefs and preconceptions still exist in some areas of the health system: more is better; it is better if it is more expensive or more specialized and high tech; it is better to do something than nothing or to wait; and better sooner than later. Pervasive incentives tend to reinforce these beliefs. Mammography screening, prostate antigen testing and genetic testing are often overused or inappropriately used. While they may be effective in certain circumstances, more is not necessarily better and may even be inappropriate. Perceptions and beliefs grounded on inaccurate information can have serious consequences.

Lag time in diffusion and uptake of information

The *Ottawa Ankle Rules* is an example of good evidence that has not reached all practices due to lag time in diffusion and uptake of

evidence by practitioners, particularly those in small or geographically remote areas. The *Ottawa Ankle Rules* represents scientifically sound, stable and generally applicable evidence, and use of the rules is considered safe, effective and efficient.

This example illustrates the need to improve the diffusion and uptake of information as evidence becomes available.

Ankle and foot injuries are common complaints among patients in emergency departments. Though only a few of these cases have suffered a fracture, nearly all undergo radiography. To address this clinical problem, the Ottawa Ankle Rules *was developed in 1992 as a non-radiological assessment tool for ankle injuries. The Rules, based on assessment of the ability to bear weight and areas of bone tenderness, allows physicians to determine quickly which patients are at negligible risk of fracture. In pilot projects, use of the rules over a prolonged period by physicians of varying experience led to a decrease in ankle radiography, waiting times and costs without an increase in missed fractures (Stiell et al., 1995).*

Overwhelming amounts of information

The pace of research in medicine and biology over the last two decades has been challenging for those attempting to synthesize and apply even a portion of what is produced. In some instances, the quantity of information is over-whelming. The British Medical Association has estimated that two million medical articles are published each year. General practitioners would need to read 19 articles a day, 365 days a year to keep up with the developments in their own practice (Radford, 1995). Rarely do users have the time, skills, assistance or tools to make sense of such a vast amount of information.

In our public consultations, we found that Canadians are less concerned with the quantity of information available than they are with the ability to get the right message to the right people at the right time. More user-friendly information and more detailed individualized information about health status and treatment choices is a common theme and request.

Decisions made without consideration of health outcomes

Historically, whether or not information was available, many health care decisions were made without explicit health outcomes in mind. For example, the construction of hospitals in the early 1980s was driven by political and employment objectives, rather than by health outcomes.

Another example is the case of drug patents. Pharmaceutical manufacturers claimed that legislation was required to adequately defend intellectual property rights. Some legislators, as well as Canada's international trade part-ners, supported the new patent legislation on the promise of increased research and devel-opment plus job creation in Canada. In

February 1993, Bill C-91 (Patent Act Amendment Act, 1992) was passed eliminat-ing compulsory licensing.[1] A number of studies estimated the cost. The federal government calculated that costs would increase by $129 million over the five years from 1992 to 1996. The government of Ontario estimated that, over 10 years, costs would increase by as much as $1 billion. Calculations of this kind require innumerable assumptions and are notoriously hard to compute. A range of esti-mates is common. A study by a professor of pharmaceutical economics at the University of Minnesota, for instance, estimated that Bill C-91 would cost taxpayers between $3.6 and $7.3 billion in constant dollars by the year 2010 (Price Waterhouse, 1996). While the financial burden of this legislative change on the pharmaceutical user and the health care sector is difficult to calculate, it is clear that the decision favoured the interests of large corporations and pharmaceutical manufacturers rather than users.

Informed stakeholders have little patience for decision makers who neither articulate clearly nor make the basis for their decisions transpar-ent, especially when these decisions affect health and health care. During one consulta-tion, members of the public and stakeholders expressed the view that they might concur with decisions being taken if they were privy to the rationale underlying the decision. They believe that the tight fiscal climate demands more accountability and that decisions affect-ing health and health care must make explicit the evidence that was used — or not used — in arriving at the final outcome.

1 *Compulsary licens-ing refers to the system whereby a licence was granted by the Commis-sioner of Patents permitting the licensee to import, make, use or sell a patented invention pertaining to a medicine. Drug manufacturers granted a licence would pay royalties (determined by the Commissioner) to the holder of the patent. Bill C-91 abolished Canada's innovative compul-sory licensing sys-tem, effectively extended the brand name companies' monopoly and ensured that a brand name prod-uct would be pro-tected from generic competition until the patents on the products had expired.*

Private industry can also influence health and health care decisions and the uptake of evidence. Advertising and the industrial clout of large organizations often drive decisions and actions on products, such as drugs, cigarettes and alcohol, which are detrimental to healthy behaviours and increase health care costs. Private industry also has an enormous influence on the dissemination of information and adoption of new interventions. For example, genetic testing and certain health care technologies have been aggressively and effectively marketed by private manufacturers.

Differing and changing values

Society in general, including the health sector, has come through a period where we believed that it was better to do more than less and something rather than nothing. As a result many decisions have been, and continue to be, made disregarding available evidence. Individual self-interest, values, beliefs, emotions and other factors often drive the process, and the lack of shared interests and values results in poor decisions and outcomes.

There is some evidence that beliefs and behaviour can be changed with appropriate information and tools. Benign prostatic hyperplasia (BPH) provides one example of how incorporating best available evidence into treatment guidelines and tools allows patients to get information and become more involved in making decisions about their health and health care. The guidelines can be combined with a decision support tool (such as an interactive video) to help both provider and patient select the most appropriate treatment. They

describe the condition itself and the relative benefits and harms associated with invasive and non-invasive treatment choices.

Many patients who have used the decision support tool choose a regimen of watchful waiting rather than more active and invasive treatments such as prostatectomy, since BPH is rarely life threatening. Evaluation of this tool demonstrates that patients using it have an improved knowledge of risks, benefits, symptoms and treatment options. More such guidelines and tools are needed to support patients in making informed choices.

Lack of accountability

Applying best evidence in the decision-making process can result in more positive health and health care outcomes and greater accountability. When decisions are made without best available information, less than optimal health and health care outcomes result. Stakeholder surveys and cost evaluations are rarely conducted or applied. Furthermore, the discipline of using resources wisely is not applied rigorously by all decision makers.

We recognize that accountability for some decisions is influenced by the fact that many population health strategies have a long lag time before positive outcomes are achieved. There will not always be a direct link between services provided today and ultimate health outcomes. For example, due to the 20-year lag time between implementation of preventive measures to reduce smoking rates and any decrease in the number of smoking-related illnesses and deaths, we cannot rely on intermediate indicators to measure their effectiveness. The outcome is not measured by current rates of smoking but rather by a decline in smoking-related morbidity and mortality, which can only be measured over a number of years.

Tradition and judgment

For centuries, providers have based treatments more on judgment than on scientific evidence. People got sick and providers would try different interventions to determine which one worked best for a given individual under certain circumstances. If a particular practice appeared beneficial, it often became the treatment or intervention of choice among providers. Even today, where evidence has conclusively shown the ineffectiveness of specific interventions, some of these interventions are still in use.

We believe that professional judgment itself can be a barrier to improving overall accountability for decision outcomes or used as a shield against using available evidence. Some decision makers use the mystical nature of medicine or administrative health care decision making to shield themselves from review and evaluation.

The practice of medicine will always rely on a certain amount of clinical judgment, which should not be replaced, but rather complemented with good evidence. It is our opinion that one cannot exist without the other. Although tolerable ranges of practice variations are acceptable, the goal is to see judgments converging to achieve comparable and best possible practice outcomes. Wide ranging

judgment is narrowed by skilled physicians using evidence. We need to ask questions of providers who are outside justifiable ranges of practice.

Privacy and confidentiality of information

Person-specific information is one of the key requirements for the development of a health information system. Protecting the confidentiality of individual health information is also critical and deserves high priority. Unless safeguards are found to protect individual health information, the need for privacy, security and confidentiality remains a huge barrier to the development of a Canadian health information system.

Person-specific information is one of the key requirements for the development of a health information system.

At the same time, better access to personal and private information can improve the decisions of health care professionals. Participants in Forum consultations told us that doctors and their patients benefit from access to more complete patient information currently scattered about in hospitals, agencies and other branches of government such as social services. In emergency situations, getting information about patient problems and treatment regimens may save lives.

Access to health information and administrative data by health researchers can also benefit society. Linking different data sets provides an opportunity to improve our understanding of the relationship between the many determinants of population health. Access to employment data and links to health data allow researchers to investigate the health effects of unemployment. Access to the demographic statistics of patients can lead to a better understanding of specific health problems across the nation and to more effective and targeted health interventions. Each of these opportunities for further research poses a challenge for decision makers to resolve the tension between the research agenda and the importance of confidentiality of personal information. Research initiatives which protect privacy and provide useful information to benefit society should be encouraged.

Information is often inappropriately managed because of professional turf wars, fear of breaching confidentiality and general lack of understanding of the management of personal and research information. As well, due to the overwhelming rate of production of information and rapid advances in health information systems and technology, the public has told us that their trust in governments, researchers and institutions in protecting their personal information has eroded. To support an evidence-based health system, public trust must be restored. Guidelines are needed for information management relevant to the various sources of information including patient health records and research.

While we need adequate protection of privacy and confidentiality, we must also recognize that there are many users of information systems, and that consumers and providers are motivated by different incentives than those that stimulate commercial interests.

Many believe that the research community should be exempt from legislation governing the use of data in the commercial sphere. We are not aware of any circumstances in Canada in which researchers have released data with pernicious or profit-oriented intent. Legislation that protects data, regardless of the user's intention, threatens to block a number of research projects. Scientists and health policy professionals depend on links to a number of information sources, over a long time, to determine causality between the life we lead and the morbidity we endure.

Canada's Privacy Commissioner (1996) acknowledges the trade-off between the uses of aggregated and integrated data and the risks to an individual's privacy. Individuals must be assured that health statistics will contribute to the overall well-being of Canadians. Corporate interests should not profit from data compiled in the public interest. The public cannot, however, rely solely on technology, including access codes and masked identifiers, to secure privacy. We are not aware of any computer system which is entirely safe from hackers— the weakest link is the authorized users.

Participants during public consultations expressed varying levels of concern for confidentiality of individual health information. They identified the urgent need to better inform the public and health care providers on the differences between personal data and data stripped of personal identifiers, aggregate information, the regulatory processes for data including ownership and access, the various uses of health information and the importance of research and subject participation.

The need for informed consent by individuals for disclosure of their personal medical records, ethical screening of research proposals and data ownership by individuals or communities in appropriate circumstances were also recognized as priorities. Greater public understanding of the issue will build trust and facilitate solutions which balance respect for individual privacy and benefits to society from research using personal health information.

Uncoordinated development of health information systems

The current health information system, while providing a wealth of population-based information in Canada, is built on a system of separate health sectors and information systems. For example, data regarding mental health, long-term care and hospitals are collected and analyzed separately. As a result many of these data are neither standardized nor intergrated.

A strategy must be identified to define uniformly, and standardize collection methods across provinces to enable nation-wide comparisons of data and information. The hospital financial data base is one example of useful comparable information which has been collected using a standardized method.

Data sets must become more comprehensive and integrated to include other health indicators and intersectoral data. To coordinate the health information system and improve decision making using best evidence, we need better application of current information, improvement in broader-based health information systems and more focused disease prevention and control surveillance systems.

New and expanded health information systems must have an integrated population-based focus linking data on the health of populations to data on health determinants, including health care usage, service expenditures in various sectors and the capacity of various sectors. Information must be evaluated in terms of relevance and its relationship to outcomes. Data must be standardized and linkages created between systems. This will require a more coordinated approach to future health information system developments.

The Canadian Network for the Advancement of Research, Industry and Education (CANARIE) and the Information Highway Advisory Council (IHAC) have undertaken to define a vision for an integrated Canadian health information infrastructure. They have articulated the need for a coordinated and integrated approach, and developed recommendations for achieving this vision (CANARIE, 1996; Industry Canada,1995).

On this subject, CANARIE released its report *Towards a Canadian Health Iway: Vision, Opportunities and Future Steps*. CANARIE intends to accelerate discussions among potential stakeholders and other public and private sector organizations in Canada leading to the development of a *Canadian Health Iway*, envisioned as a network of networks, applications and people that collectively support a wide range of health-related systems, activities and services in support of Canadians in all parts of Canada. Each application envisaged for the *Health Iway* would require investment in the development of appropriate data bases, user interfaces and retrieval and decision support mechanisms.

The final report of Industry Canada's Information Highway Advisory Committee (IHAC), *Connection, Community, Content: The Challenge of the Information Highway*, supporting the building of a health information infrastructure, recommends convening "a working group of all stakeholders to address the challenges of implementing a health information infrastructure and to identify applications that would benefit all Canadians; and creating an investment fund to support demonstrations of networking technology of specific benefit to the health sector and communities at large."

How Do We Know That We Need to Improve the Use of Evidence?

Ontario's Institute for Clinical Evaluative Sciences *(ICES) Practice Atlas* (1996) and the British Columbia *Provincial Health Officer's Annual Report* (1996) are two reports published in Canada which document variations in practice patterns, suggesting that evidence is not used uniformly in the provision of services. These are only the latest in a large collection of similar studies in many countries, extending over the last 30 years. Rarely have these studies elicited any systematic response.

A case in point is the rate of Cesarean sections. The Cesarean section rate in Canada increased steadily from about six percent of deliveries in the early 1970s to 20 percent in the mid-1980s and then declined slightly to 17 percent in 1994-1995. Since the mid-1980s, lower rates have been promoted but in many areas they remain high. Cesarean section rates vary considerably between provinces, within provinces and between hospitals (ICES, 1996). In British Columbia, 1994 statistics indicated that the difference between the lowest and highest hospital rates was close to threefold, with rates ranging from 10 to 29 percent of births (British Columbia Provincial Health Officer, 1996). Research suggests that only 10 to 12 percent of pregnancies require Cesarean deliveries (Joffe et al., 1994; Helewa, 1995).

Practice variations also occur for surgical treatment of benign prostatic hyperplasia

(BPH). Some providers have questioned the usefulness of the evidence to support clinical practice (Tranmer et al., 1997). Physicians claim that multiple guidelines exist and that evidence is confusing and conflicting. Cost effectiveness of watchful waiting is questioned by some providers who imply that extra testing and drug prescriptions may be just as costly as surgical intervention. These providers are demanding more conclusive information to convince them that a practice change is best for both the patient and the overall health system. They place the onus on the researchers to provide sound and compelling evidence which will convince them to change practice standards.

Variations in practice may also be linked to economic conditions that threaten income. In the case of BPH, there is an economic disincentive for some physicians to adopt best evidence which might point to a reduced need for surgical intervention and thus a related reduction in income. As well, economic conditions strongly influence administration and policy. For example, hospital bed reductions and closures are swayed by threats to employment and income.

We believe that the generation of enough compelling evidence, coupled with incentives and greater public accountability, will change all practice patterns so that they fall within acceptable ranges of variation. Quality evidence and wisdom applied to all decisions at all levels —- policy and regulation, management and administration and in clinical settings are key to improving health care and outcomes.

Signs of Progress

Despite the varying quantity and quality of available evidence and the complexities of its use, good evidence does exist and is being used. Improvements are encouraging the production and use of more good information.

The activities and initiatives of many organizations in Canada are going a long way toward making evidence more available, accessible and usable to decision makers in our health system. Some of this activity originated over 20 years ago and evolved with the development of the health and health care system. In research, national granting councils and programs such as the Medical Research Council, the National Health Research and Development Program and the Social Sciences and Humanities Research Council are complemented by a number of provincially based and philanthropic research granting bodies (Alberta Heritage Foundation, Heart and Stroke Foundation).

Improvements are encouraging the production and use of more good information.

Some organizations are involved in developing practice guidelines and assessing the use of clinical tools by conducting systematic reviews of published research data. For example, the Canadian Task Force on the Periodic Health Examination, a highly regarded group, reviews the literature on controlled trials and epidemiological studies. It grades each intervention on whether or not the evidence justifies continuation of the intervention which may refer to a variety of tests, examinations, and counselling on apparently healthy individuals. There should be provincial monitoring to determine if its recommendations are being followed and to question practice variation patterns. The Canadian Medical Association is also a main player in clinical practice guideline development.

The Canadian Coordinating Office for Health Technology Assessment (CCOHTA) encourages appropriate use of health technology through the collection, analysis and dissemination of information concerning the effectiveness and cost of technology and its impact on health. The methodology is to review randomized controlled trials from international researchers and to incorporate other evidence, including economic evaluations, when appropriate. The Canadian Cochrane Collaboration assesses clinical trials to advance clinical knowledge on the appropriateness of alternative medical interventions.

A larger number of national and provincial organizations are involved in standardizing, collecting, analyzing and reporting individual and population health information. The Canadian Institute for Health Information among other functions, maintains a data base for hospital discharge information used by health care institutions and provincial ministries. The Manitoba Centre for Health Policy and Evaluation has the Populis data base which is used to describe and explain patterns of care and profiles of health and illness. It analyzes administrative data collected by the provincial health insurance system and documents every patient contact made with hospitals, nursing homes and physicians in the

province. These data have been used to assess the impact of closing 20 percent of Winnipeg's acute care hospital beds on the public's access and quality of care, and health of the population (Brownell and Roos, 1996). These data are also being used to compare costs in different hospitals and to develop performance indicators. Statistics Canada, the Institute for Clinical and Evaluative Sciences in Ontario, Med-Echo in Quebec, and probably others, are involved in similar activities.

At the federal and provincial level, population health surveys are carried out at varying intervals. The last national population health survey was conducted by Statistics Canada in 1994 in collaboration with provinces and territories.

A few organizations concentrate on health services and policy issues: the Saskatchewan Health Services Utilization Review Commission, the Centre for Health Economics and Policy Analysis, the University of British Columbia Centre for Health Policy, the *Université de Montréal groupe de recherche interdisciplinaire en santé (GRIS)* and the Queen's Health Policy Unit to name a few.

There are also health surveillance activities in Health Canada and provincial departments of health which generate a significant amount of information on diseases, pathogens and modes of transmission.

Some organizations focus on health concerns of particular groups using data produced by someone else: the Canadian Institute for Child

Health, the Canadian Association for School Health, etc. Yet others have interests in only one component of the health care system and are developing systems designed to capture and use data in that area: Pharmanet is one example. Another example is the National Student/Child School/Community Feeding Program Research Network which, in pursuing research work on the effectiveness of school nutrition programs, determined that the first task was the development of a national data base on these programs. There are also groups working on the development of commercial applications of research findings. HealNet is a network of such groups, brought together with federal funding.

Many national health organizations focusing on specific diseases or health concerns (cancer, arthritis, diabetes, kidney disease, heart and stroke, Alzheimer's disease, etc) provide information to consumers on appropriate treatment or sources of help and information. Consumers also turn to libraries and the Internet in search of information on health matters. Some clinical practice guidelines are available on the Internet as a doctor's version and in a shorter version intended for the public. As well, news groups on health topics and on specific diseases and conditions are accessible on the Internet, and new ones are formed every day.

Most health information initiatives have international connections. In fact, a good number of them for (example, Cochrane, CCOHTA, most academic institutes) could not survive without such connections. While people in all of these organizations or units probably know of each other and read each other's publica-

tions, there is no systematic integrated plan to link their work nor is there a clear sense of possible gaps which exist between them. They, nevertheless, constitute an immense resource and represent a considerable investment on which we believe we must build.

We endorse these initiatives and seek ways to improve information capacity in Canada and to foster a culture of evidence-based decision making.

During a period of change, people value evidence to anchor their decisions, to validate their choices. Quality information and evidence is comforting, especially when decisions are complex and tough. But there are other reasons for creating an evidence-based health system, and there are questions yet to be answered.

Achieving the Vision

The vision of an evidence-based health system requires a number of things: quantitative and qualitative evidence, linked and integrated information systems and technology, tools that promote diffusion and uptake of information and incentives to change behaviour. Information gaps must be addressed concerning women's health issues, gender-appropriate research, alternative and complementary interventions and non-medical determinants of health.

The concept of evidence-based decision making must be championed by credible leaders throughout the system. Explicit support for its broadened use must be evident from top policy makers, to providers and administrators and to users of health services.

As part of the vision for an evidence-based culture, universal access to requisite information and the know-how to use the information, technology and tools should be priority objectives. Bold new initiatives must be found to improve the understanding and capabilities of the information and technology at hand and the knowledge to use this available information to help make better decisions.

To broaden the use of information, one focus must be on improving access. The technology gap between rich and poor Canadians is widening where there is not a systematic approach to ensure equitable access (Industry Canada, 1995). Access to and proficiency with computer technology are concentrated among high-income, well-educated Canadians. For example, more than 50 percent of households with incomes in excess of $70,000 have home computers compared with 11 percent of households with incomes below $15,000. (Oderkirk, 1996). People who are unemployed or who have little education face the possibility of becoming further marginalized as other Canadians use computers to acquire new knowledge. Special efforts must be made to identify the gaps and direct resources to the have-nots. Many suggest that such efforts should be targeted to schools. For example, SchoolNet[2] aims to have Canada's 23,000 schools and libraries connected to the Internet by 1998. In the development of linked health systems and technology, there is opportunity to equalize the access and capabilities of those individuals who have the technology and knowledge to use it, and those who do not.

Although much more research and work needs to be done on the actual impact of strategies for integrating information into practice, the participation of local opinion leaders, a reminder and feedback system, and incentives to reorganize the allocation of resources within practice and policy are three major factors in changing behaviour.

The public can play a major role in creating this culture. By arming themselves with the information, mobilizing their interests and influencing health policy, Canadians will challenge the status quo. Decision makers will respond by becoming more accountable.

A better informed public will influence evidence-based decision making. Governments should lead the way in strengthening public and user influence to create this culture.

More informed and involved users will lead to better health care decisions and accountability.

---

2 *SchoolNet is a cooperative venture by federal and provincial governments.*

Some people spend considerable energy in acquiring information before making major purchases or in making arrangements for their children's education and day care. We must assist the public to become more discriminating about health care. Recognizing that the public and the patient do not always want to be involved in decision making, creating opportunities will encourage more public and patient involvement where it is desired.

Public influence is only one factor which affects use of information. It is also affected by individual characteristics of the decision maker, organizational structures and processes, economic, social and regulatory environments within which the organization or decision maker exist, and the quality, relevance and presentation of the information.

Tools and incentives are needed to encourage understanding and use of best available information in the decision-making process. They must be developed and incorporated into daily operation of services and provide feedback on performance and consequences of decisions. These tools must facilitate and improve professional practice, and value-added benefits of their acceptance must be demonstrated. For example, including at the point of service an automated prescribing system for clinicians would provide relevant, accurate information on drugs and their uses, contraindications and side effects. With input on patient characteristics, the system would recommend treatment options based on best available evidence. The physician has the option to apply experience and judgment to individual circumstance and override the best available evidence, but not without feedback. The value-added benefit is that it saves the clinician the time needed to

research the information and also provides automatic transfers of prescriptions to the dispensing pharmacist as well as administrative information for payment purposes.

Our health system is complex, and creating an evidence-based culture remains a great challenge. Three key ingredients must be present. The first is timely availability of evidence for all decision makers. The second is uptake of information with appropriate incentives, methods and tools to ensure use. The third is accountability of decision makers and performance feedback.

More informed and involved users will lead to better health care decisions and accountability.

One firm conclusion of our work is that Canada must move quickly toward an evidence-based health system if Canada's premier social program is to be preserved. Progress towards the development of a nationwide health information system must continue to produce the intelligence and knowledge required. If progress is delayed, evidence is unlikely to be the basis on which decisions are made, and we will lose the opportunity to make the system more efficient and more effective, throwing the future of the health system into jeopardy.

One overriding recommendation, therefore, is that Canada move rapidly toward the development of an evidence-based health system and put in place the resources required to achieve this goal.

The following recommendations support and enable the attainment of this major objective.

Leadership

The development of an evidence-based health system requires political will, leadership and champions. The foundation of an evidence-based health system must be a health information system capable of operating at both the provincial/territorial and national levels, and that provides value-added, comparative information for provinces/territories, regions and sub-populations.

We need to identify what we want in a Canadian health information system and agree on a vision for its further development. Until we do, more investments in health information systems may risk becoming obstacles in building an integrated, coordinated and interconnected system.

We recommend that:

a) The federal Minister of Health champion the creation of an evidence-based health system, built on the foundation of a national health information system. This active leadership role requires collaboration with both provincial and territorial health ministers and other federal departments.

b) In addition, this leadership role include the establishment of a number of time-limited stakeholder groups drawn from provincial and territorial governments, providers, industry, researchers and the public to undertake tasks necessary for creating an evidence-based health system.

Improving Public Accountability Through a Nation-wide Health Information System

A nation-wide health information system must be created which goes beyond data warehousing to create different levels of information to support clinical, policy and health services decision making as well as decision making by the patient and public at large. Such information has potential to:

- help make better decisions which improve population health;

- achieve greater efficiency in the expenditure of health care resources; and

- improve accountability for positive health outcomes.

The system must provide information to answer such questions as:

- Is the health of the population poor in an area because of lack of access to health care, or despite good access to health care?

- Are expenditures high in some areas in congruence with residents at high risk for poor health or simply because the area has excess hospital capacity despite the good health of area residents?

- Are there differences in cost effectiveness of some services in one area compared to another?

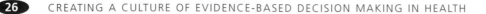

It is essential that the system link socioeconomic determinants of health, personal behaviours that influence health, usage of health care resources, supply and capacity of the health care system and expenditures on health care so that better decisions can be made. Comprehensive comparative national information should be available that focuses on vulnerable populations such as children, Aboriginal peoples and persons living in poverty.

The National Task Force on Health Information (1991) presented comprehensive goals and a strong vision for a nation-wide health information system. The Task Force identified several functions needed to ensure public accountability: collecting and analyzing information, reporting to the public on health status and health system performance, promoting the need for population health research and evidence-based decision making, and developing and responding to health policy. The Task Force also acknowledged that the development of a nation-wide health information system requires cooperation and partnerships.

While many of the Task Force goals have been met, some have not yet been achieved. There is, therefore, a significant gap. Specifically, some of the many functions needed to ensure public accountability are not being fulfilled. As currently constituted, no current organization has the capacity to carry out all of these functions.

We believe that the vision of the National Task Force on Health Information remains valid today. We concur that a nation-wide network of provincial, territorial and national

agencies is needed to implement this vision. The provincial/territorial agencies should have a mandate to develop and maintain a standardized set of longitudinal data on health status and health system performance, which would make up the components of a national population health data system. They should also be mandated to advocate for, and advance the population health agenda. They should report to the public annually on key trends, significant inter- and intra-provincial comparisons, and relevant public policy issues arising from such analysis.

Within that network, a central national agency is needed which we would refer to as a "National Population Health Institute." This agency would have the following functions within its mandate: aggregate and analyze data collected by the provincial/territorial and other agencies, coordinate the development of data standards, report to the public on national health status and health system performance, promote research and the use of evidence in decision making, and act as a resource for the development and evaluation of public policy. It would collaborate with provincial and territorial agencies in advocating for and advancing the population health agenda. The National Population Health Institute would also report publicly on national trends, international and interprovincial comparisons and key public policy issues.

These agencies need to be governed and funded in ways that preserve their credibility and independence from government as well as from users of their services, data and reports. Multi-year funding is required to maintain stability and credibility. The structure of the national agency, to be effective, should include provincial, territorial and academic involvement.

Such agencies exist in a few provinces but not in all. At the national level, the Canadian Institute for Health Information was established in 1994 pursuant to the adoption, by the conference of ministers of health, of the report of the National Task Force on Health Information. We are aware of the agencies currently in existence and believe that they should be taken into account in the implementation of our recommendations.

We recommend that:

a) *A national population health data network be established linking provincial, territorial agencies and a national agency. In creating this network, the federal/provincial/ territorial ministers of health must ensure that issues and barriers confronting this initiative such as privacy, security and confidentiality, standards (technical as well as operational), and funding for research and development are addressed and consensus on a national development and implementation plan is established.*

b) *Provincial/territorial agencies be mandated to develop and maintain a standardized set of longitudinal data on health status and health system performance and to advocate for, and advance the population health agenda.*

c) *A National Population Health Institute be put in place as soon as possible with a mandate to aggregate and analyze data, develop data standards and common definitions, report to the public on national overall health status and health system performance and act as a resource for the development and evaluation of public policy. The National Population Health Institute would collaborate with provincial and territorial agencies. It would also report publicly on national trends, international and interprovincial comparisons and key public policy issues.*

d) *Governance and funding arrangements for the agencies in the network be adequately balanced to preserve their credibility and independence and be sufficiently secure over time to ensure their stability. The national agency structure should have provincial, territorial and academic involvement.*

e) *For purposes of establishing the National Population Health Institute, the mandate, organization and funding of existing agencies, particularly the Canadian Institute of Health Information, be reviewed without delay to ascertain whether any of them could fulfil the recommended mandate effectively. If that is not possible, a new agency must be created. Where applicable in provinces and territories, similar evaluations should be performed.*

To illustrate potential usefulness of a more coherent and linked health information system, one of the first steps could be the production of a Health and Health Care Atlas.

The Atlas should:

■ use existing sources of information;

■ compare the Canadian population across meaningful, provincially defined geographic areas; and

■ link data on health status, factors influencing the need for health care, patterns of health care use, and supply of health care services.

Research and Evaluation

Research plays a critical role in the development of quality content for a nation-wide health information system. We know that overwhelming amounts of evidence currently exist and that evidence is continually changing, and is often confusing and conflicting. Research must respond by developing and applying assessment and synthesis methods that are appropriate for multi-disciplinary sources of evidence; and by addressing information gaps, particularly in non-medical determinants of health, gender-specific research, women's health issues, and complementary and alternative interventions. Research must be conducted using methodologies that are appropriate to gender and culture. Research designs should be appropriate to population groups, ensure privacy of the participants and provide information that benefits society at large.

Synthesis of existing information which addresses women's health issues has to be a priority for the research agenda. Women earn less. Women predominantly inhabit lower levels of the occupational hierarchy. And women tend to have less control over their work situation. There are not enough female researchers to promote women's health, nor are there enough women enrolled in clinical trials and other research initiatives to define risks and benefits of interventions, technologies and drug therapies for women. Women must be assured that interventions applied to them are appropriate and effective. Public policies, similarly, have a different impact on women and men. For example, if we shift from institutional care to community-based services without increasing public funding for these services, we have to recognize that we are also shifting additional responsibility to women who are the primary care givers in most families. It is crucial that the mental, social and physical health and well-being concerns unique to women climb to a prominent position on the health research and funding agenda.

The safety and effectiveness of alternative interventions also requires urgent attention. Currently, we have little information to help assess which interventions are beneficial (or potentially harmful). With the growing public interest in alternative therapies and treatment choices, it is imperative that assessment and evaluation of existing therapies are undertaken. New research on alternative therapies should also be a priority.

Research on Aboriginal health issues is a paramount need. While existing evidence indicates that the health status of Aboriginal peoples is poor in comparison to the general Canadian population, information is lacking on effective culturally-specific interventions to improve the health status of Aboriginal peoples.

The emerging perspectives on population health and its determinants emphasize the need to review the information and understand the impact of non-medical interventions on population health status. The knowledge base concerning the social, economic and cultural determinants of health and the efficacy of non-medical interventions is weak in comparison with our knowledge of medical determinants of health.

We recommend that:

A time-limited stakeholder group, under the leadership of the federal/provincial/territorial ministers of health, consider the following components in the development of a research agenda:

a) *Undertaking a strategic overview of current state of health-related knowledge — what we know, what we don't know, and what we need to know to support the efficient and effective management of the health and health care sector. Gaps in our current knowledge and areas where there is a paucity of research, analysis and translation, such as in the non-medical determinants of health, gender-specific health outcomes, women's health issues, Aboriginal health issues and alternative and complementary practices, must be identified.*

b) *Identifying the best mechanisms for promoting synthesis, translation, dissemination and uptake of existing information into useful knowledge where primary research data are already available. The potential role of information technology in these activities needs to be explored.*

Funding

Governments should continue to support research funding. Offloading of research costs to the private sector will be a major obstacle to improving effective management of research needs and priorities. Private industry budgets, including pharmaceutical research, are large and very influential. Furthermore, private spending on research and development sets a certain direction and is generally intended to develop new marketable products, which may distort the broader research agenda.

Recognition of the need for synthesized high-quality information and for research on information gaps and emerging issues is relatively new. Health research funding must move toward a more appropriate balance between research into non-medical and medical health determinants.

Funding must be secured to fulfil the research agenda and the human resource development requirements. To support these new research priorities and enable translation of information into user-friendly support tools, specific skill sets and training are needed.

The health sector, in its reform process, has displaced many health workers who remain unemployed. The development of health information requires a number of individuals with skills and knowledge in health as well as in information and networking technologies. There would be considerable benefits and savings in human resources if we could offer successful retraining opportunities for unemployed health workers to acquire these needed skills.

CANARIE's TAD (Technology Application Development) Program, in targeting health applications, has created opportunities to fund developments in information technology in the health sector. A recent announcement of a new initiative by Industry Canada, called Technology Partnerships Canada (TPC) also provides opportunities for the development of the information highway in the health sector. The focus of both programs is on economic development and strategies to promote private sector competitiveness. Initial funding decisions have, therefore, supported the development of the physical infrastructure, with less on applications and almost nothing in the development of content. The development of the health information system requires the generation of content, applications and the physical infrastructure connecting the "last mile" to health centres, offices and homes. This requires a funding approach different from that which currently exists.

The Health Services Research Fund, created in 1996, is a potential source of funding but we acknowledge that there will be many worthy initiatives competing for these resources. Another potential funding source is the Canada Infrastructure Works Program[3] to support development of the information highway in the public sector — in health, education and government services. The program could complement other sources of funding and provide opportunities for unemployed health care workers to acquire new skills needed for the information society.

---

3. *Canada Infrastructure Works is a $6 billion program designed to renew Canada's infrastructure and generate employment. In 1995, the program was extended from three to five years and will run until 1998/99 fiscal year. Costs are shared equally by the federal, provincial and municipal governments. While the majority of approved projects are for roads, highways, bridges, water systems, sewers and other municipal buildings such as fire stations, there are a number of projects which are developing and enhancing information systems and technology.*

We recommend that:

A stakeholder group reporting to the federal/provincial/territorial ministers of health identify:

a) *Potential funding opportunities for development of the nation-wide health information system including applications, content and physical infrastructure needs.*

b) *Requirements for funding human resource development.*

c) *Strategies for shifting funding emphasis to create an appropriate balance between research on non-medical determinants and basic and clinical sciences research, with emphasis on career support funding, and equal emphasis on investigator-initiated and policy-relevant allotments.*

Improving Dissemination and Uptake of Evidence

The best available information is worthless if it is not used or is disregarded when decisions are being made. To promote the uptake of evidence, we must understand the factors and opportunities which influence its adoption as well as the major barriers which hinder it.

Economic conditions and financial factors can be strong barriers to the uptake and use of evidence. Alternatively, they may be powerful incentives for their use. Some forms of remuneration work better than others in encouraging the most cost-effective interventions. Therefore, funding and remuneration systems should be matched with services and programs to enable and facilitate practice and policy changes if indicated by best available information.

Other incentives, as well as automated and non-automated tools which help put evidence into use, must be developed to address the different needs of many decision makers. They should all provide value-added benefits to the user. Decision makers need to know that these incentives and tools will make their work and decisions easier and improve their accountability and above all, improve the quality of health outcomes. If information is believed to be useful, it will be used.

A number of non-economic incentives and strategies, such as clinical practice guidelines, consensus reports, practice variation analyses and decision support tools, have been developed in efforts to encourage adoption of best evidence into health care practice and policy. These tools and incentives must be evidence driven and grounded in examination of real practice patterns. They must explicitly provide evidence reflecting both what decision makers actually do, compared against benchmarks and the difference in health care outcomes when best evidence is used. They must provide high-quality information and performance feedback, and offer the decision maker value-added benefits if they are to be effective.

We recommend that:

a) A time-limited stakeholder group, under the leadership of the federal/provincial/territorial ministers of health, identify strategies which support the continued development of incentives and methods that improve the dissemination and adoption of health information into best practice and policy.

b) Experiments which examine how modification of tools or complementary initiatives can improve the adoption of evidence be encouraged. The Transition Fund proposed by the National Forum on Health is one method to pursue these experiments.

c) Initiatives for integrating evidence-based decision making tools into professional practice to support the uptake of information and, where indicated, practice or policy change be supported.

d) Licensing bodies incorporate the use and development of evidence-based clinical practice guidelines into standards of care required of members. These guidelines must be widely distributed and disseminated to all members.

e) Funders of health services (provincial/territorial governments and regional health bodies) adopt funding models, such as budgetary envelopes, with service providers to encourage the use of best practices.

Balancing Privacy and Accessibility of Health Information

The Medical Research Council, the Natural Sciences and Engineering Research Council and the Social Sciences and Humanities Research Council are committed to supporting and supervising the quest for improved medical and social interventions. The Tri-Council Committee, comprised of these three granting councils, produced a Code of Conduct for Research Involving Humans. The councils support development of a single set of privacy and confidentiality rules that would apply to the research community as well as to commercial and governmental interests.

The basic principle of the Tri-Council is to find a workable balance between the protection of the interests of individuals and groups and the promotion of research that will enhance our knowledge of the determinants of the well-being of these individuals and groups. The Code of Conduct is a non-binding document that devolves responsibility for monitoring adherence to its principles to institution-based research ethics boards.

The Tri-Council Code relies on voluntary codes of compliance, but there are objections to this from other arms of the government. The federal Privacy Commissioner cautions that having the private sector opt in to voluntary privacy codes is a grossly inadequate assurance in return for gaining access to data and transactions which now have legal protection (Privacy Commissioner of Canada, 1996).

We endorse the Tri-Council principle for balance between the strict protection of the interests of individuals and the promotion of public good through research.

We recommend that:

a) *Where plans for model legislation proceed, the ministers of Justice and Industry, in preparing proposals for the protection of personal data in the private sector, recognize that the interest of commercial bodies in data may differ significantly from the public interest in research. While it is difficult to separate the interests of these two bodies completely, we recognize that they are distinct worlds. Risks of disclosure exist in both but the incentives are different. Legislation should protect the privacy of individuals without jeopardizing the potential benefits which data from the information system can provide. The legislation must:*

   i) *Distinguish between the administrative use of data which identifies individuals and statistical use of data which does not refer to the identity of specific individuals.*

   ii) *Distinguish between the use of the data to advance the public interest and its use in pursuit of a private or commercial interest.*

b) *We should follow the lead of the European Parliament in balancing privacy and access to data for health research in the public interest (including data which at one stage may be linked using individual identifiers). We should also adopt the principles identified by the European Parliament for managing data for health research:*

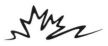

i) data collected for one purpose should not be used for another except with informed consent;

ii) information must be destroyed after a specified time period;

iii) an agency cannot disclose information to a third party unless it had been part of the stated purpose or otherwise authorized by the individual.

c) An information infrastructure be adopted which includes an access and confidentiality committee, university-based ethics committees, professional standards and clear instructions on the methods for keeping data confidential.

d) As more personal information is computerized and becomes linked and accessible to a variety of providers, privacy must be assured through safeguards such as Personal Information Identifiers (PIN).

Conclusion

Canada must move quickly toward an evidence-based health system and put into place the necessary resources to build a more effective and efficient health system. We believe that a founding element of an evidence-based health system is a health information system. If further development of a nation-wide health information system is delayed we will lose the opportunity to make the health system more effective and efficient.

A nation-wide health information system should be capable of operating at both the provincial/territorial and national levels, and provide value-added, comparative information for provinces, territories, regions and sub-populations. It must capture and link indicators of need, health status, health care and supply or system capacity. In building such an integrated and linked health information system, we must capitalize on existing strengths and partnerships, avoid duplication and unnecessary competition and progress according to a collaborative planning framework.

For success, three key ingredients must be present:

■ Enhancement of public accountability: This requires accumulation of information about population health, the medical and non-medical determinants of health and the effectiveness of health policy interventions.

■ Multi-layered high-quality content for all decision makers at all levels: This calls for ongoing research and evaluation of existing information and identification of information gaps. Emphasis must be placed on women's health issues, gender-based research, Aboriginal health issues, alternative and complementary interventions and non-medical determinants of health.

- Strategies for dissemination and uptake of information by decision makers: Financial and other incentives as well as automated and non-automated information tools are needed. Value-added benefits of using such incentives and tools must be clearly demonstrated to decision makers.

Funding sources must be identified to help build health information system capacity, link data bases, and to address implementation issues such as privacy and accessibility, and the need for standards. Funding is also needed to fulfil the research agenda. While a $65 million Health Services Research Fund exists, additional funds are needed to support the broader research priorities which include, in addition to primary data collection, the capacity for analysis, synthesis and translation of existing information, development of decision support tools and strategies for dissemination and uptake of information.

Many initiatives are already under way to improve Canada's health information capacity. The challenge will be to reach some degree of consensus on implementation issues such as data definitions and privacy of information; the development of a transitional and implementation plan; and the fill ins of any information gaps through synthesis of existing information, critical analysis and new research.

The window of opportunity is open. Canada's leaders must act now to become more fully equipped to move forward with health care reform and broader initiatives to improve the health of the population. Most important, Canadians will get the information they need in order to separate myth from reality, to challenge and ask questions about health care services and to hold decision makers accountable for the performance of the health care system and healthy public policy — in short, to become active participants in creating a more effective and efficient health system.

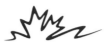

References

Baggaley, C. and D. McKendry. *The Bill C-91 Review: What are the Consumer Issues?* Price Waterhouse, September 1996.

Black, C. "Building a National Health Policy Information Network." *Papers commissioned by the National Forum on Health*. Ottawa, 1997 (in press).

British Columbia Provincial Health Officer. *A Report on the Health of British Columbians: Provincial Health Officer's Annual Report 1995*. Victoria, B.C.: Ministry of Health and Ministry Responsible for Seniors, 1996.

Brownell, M. and N. Roos. *Monitoring the Winnipeg Hospital System: the Update Report and Summary, 1993/94*. Manitoba Centre for Health Policy and Evaluation, January 1996.

Butcher, R. "Foundations for Evidence-Based Decision Making." *Papers commissioned by the National Forum on Health*. Ottawa, 1997 (in press).

Canada. Health Canada. *National Health Expenditures in Canada: 1975-94*. Ottawa, 1995.

_____. Industry Canada. *Connection, Community, Content: The Challenge of the Information Highway*. Final Report of the Information Highway Advisory Council. Ottawa, 1995.

_____. National Forum on Health. *Summary Report. Changing the Health Care System - A Consumer Perspective*. Ottawa, 1995.

_____. *Report on Dialogue with Canadians*. Ottawa, 1996.

_____. *Summary Report. Evidence-based Decision Making: A Dialogue on Health Information*. Ottawa, 1995.

Canadian Task Force on the Periodic Health Examination. *The Canadian Guide to Clinical and Preventative Health Care*. Ottawa: Health Canada, 1994.

CANARIE. *Towards a Canadian Health Iway: Vision, Opportunities and Future Steps*. 1996.

Cox, J. "Lesson in Patience and Persistence." *Nursing BC,* (Aug./Sept. 1995).

Dekkers, A. F. "Patients' Rights in the Netherlands." In *Promotion of the Rights of Patients in Europe*. Proceedings of a WHO Consultation. 1995.

Ekos Research Associates Inc. "Research on Canadian Values in Relation to Health and the Health Care System." *Papers Commissioned by the National Forum on Health*. Ottawa, 1997 (in press).

Federal, Provincial, and Territorial Advisory Committee on Population Health. *Report on the Health of Canadians*. 1996

Fisher, P., M.J. Hollander, T. MacKenzie, P. Kleinstiver, I. Sladecek and G. Peterson. "Decision Support Tools in Health Care.*" Papers Commissioned by the National Forum on Health*. Ottawa, 1997 (in press).

Godolphin, W., N. Schmitt and T.W. Anderson. "Blood Lead in Canadian Children: a Current Perspective." *Canadian Medical Association Journal*, 148 4 (1993): 517-519.

Helewa, M.E. "Caesarean Sections in Canada: What Constitutes Appropriate Rate?" *Journal of the Society of Obstetrics and Gynaecology Canada,* 17 3 (1995): 237-246.

Husten, P. "Cochrane Collaboration Helping Unravel Tangled Web Woven by International Research." *Canadian Medical Association Journal*, 154 9 (May 1).

Institute for Clinical Evaluative Sciences in Ontario (ICES). *Patterns of Health Care in Ontario. The ICES Practice Atlas*, 2nd Edition. Ottawa: Canadian Medical Association, 1996.

Joffe, M., J. Chapple, C. Patterson and R.W. Beard. "What is the Optimal Caesarian Section Rate? An Outcome Based Study of Existing Variation." *Journal of Epidemiology in Community Health*, 48 (1994): 406-411.

Judelson, D.R. "Cardiovascular disease in women." *Journal of the American Medical Women's Association*, 49 6 (1995): 180.

Kitler, M.E. "Coronary disease: Are there gender differences?" *European Heart Journal*, 15 (1994): 409-417.

Kushner, C. and M. Rachlis. "Consumer Involvement in Health Policy Development." *Papers Commissioned by the National Forum on Health*. Ottawa, 1997 (in press).

LaRosa, J.H. and L.L. Alexander. *Gender Differences: Knowns and Unknowns*. Prepared for the annual meeting of the Society for the Advancement of Research on Women's Health. Washington, D.C., 1995.

Lefebvre, Y. 1996. *Women's Health Research in Canada: A Canadian Perspective*. Canada-U.S.A. Women's Health Forum, August 1996.

Lomas, J. *Making Clinical Policy Explicit: Legislative Policy-Making and Lessons for Practice Guideline Development*. McMaster University Centre for Health Economics and Policy Analysis Working Paper # 91-12, October 1991.

_____. *Words without Action? The Production, Dissemination and Impact of Consensus Recommendations*. McMaster University Centre for Health Economics and Policy Analysis Working Paper #90-12, September 1990.

Manton, K.G. "The Dynamics of Population Aging: Demography and Policy Analysis." *The Milbank Quarterly,* 69 (1991):309-340.

McMahon T. for the ULCC Advisory Group on Protection of Personal Information. *Data Protection in the Private Sector: Options for a Uniform Statute*. Uniform Law Conference of Canada, August 1996.

Medical Research Council of Canada. *Guidelines for the Commercialization of Medical Research*, Draft Report of the Working Group on Conflict of Interest in Intellectual Property and Commercialization, February 7, 1996.

Medical Research Council of Canada, the Natural Sciences and Engineering Research Council of Canada and the Social Sciences and Humanities Research Council of Canada. *Code of Conduct for Research Involving Humans*. Prepared by the Tri-Council Working Group, March 1996.

Neilson. Overviews 03298, 03297, 032885. In *Pregnancy and Childbirth Module of Cochrane Database of Systemic Reviews*, Enkin M. Keirse, ed. Oxford: Update Software, 1994.

Oderkirk, J. 1996. "Computer Literacy - a growing requirement." *Education Quarterly Review,* 3 (3): 9-29.

Privacy Commissioner of Canada. *Annual Report 1995-96.* Ottawa, 1996.

Radford, T. *The Guardian*, p.8, Oct. 3, 1995.

Stiell, I., G. Wells, A. Laupacis, R. Brison, R. Verbeek, K. Vandemheen and C.D. Naylor. "Multicentre Trial to Introduce the Ottawa Ankle Rules for Use of Radiography in Acute Ankle Injuries." *British Medical Journal*, Vol. 311(September 2, 1995): 594-597. "Evidence-based Decision Making: What works and what doesn't work." *Papers Commissioned by the National Forum on Health*. Ottawa, 1997 (in press).

Tranmer, J. E., S. Squires, K. Brazil, J. Gerlach, J. Johnson, D. Muisner, B. Swan and R. Wilson. "Evidence-based Decision Making: What works and what doesn't work." *Papers Commissioned by the National Forum on Health*. Ottawa, 1997 (in press).

Vickey, D.M. and J. Fries. *Take Care of Yourself: A Consumer's Guide to Medical Care.* Reading, MA: Addison-Wesley Publishing Company, 1992.

Walters, K. "Alternative medicine getting mainstream recognition." *Sounding Board*. Vancouver Board of Trade, Summer 1996.

Wilk, M. *Health Information for Canada*, Report of the National Task Force on Health Information, 1991.

Wolfson, M.C., Rowe, G., Gentleman and M. Tomiak. "Career Earnings and Death: A Longitudinal Analysis of Older Canadian Men." *Journal of Gerontology: Social Sciences*, 48 4 (1993): S167-S179.

_____. "POHEM — A Framework for Understanding and Modeling the Health of Human Populations." *World Health Statistic Quarterly*, 47 3/4, Geneva: World Health Organization, 1994.

_____. "Thoughts Regarding Possible Recommendations in the Area of Health Information." Submitted to National Forum on Health, Evidence-Based Decision Making Working Group, July 1996.

Appendix 1

Overview of consultations undertaken:

Public consultations

The National Forum on Health conducted the first round (Phase I) of consultations between November 1995 and April 1996. In total, 71 discussion groups were sponsored in 34 centres across Canada on the future of the health system. Approximately 1,300 Canadians participated.

The issue of how to make good decisions about health funding, health resource allocation and medical intervention was of particular concern to the Evidence-Based Decision Making Working Group. Specifically, three questions were explored:

■ Who should decide which treatments are effective or ineffective and which treatments are appropriate or inappropriate?

■ Should more expensive treatments be publicly funded when less expensive treatments with similar effect are available?

■ Do Canadians have access to the information they require to make effective decisions about their own and their family's health care requirements?

To ensure that a diversity of Canadians participated in this process, several sessions were held in Aboriginal communities. As well, groups with special health needs, including homeless men in Toronto, new Canadians in London, street youth in Victoria and Toronto, and retired persons in Penticton met with Forum members and the Secretariat. Finally,

self-directed workbooks were mailed out to others who wished to participate in this process and express their views but who were unable to attend the scheduled regional discussion groups.

The second round (Phase II) of consultations was held between October 1996 and November 1996. The Forum held two national conferences, in Vancouver and Montreal, and commissioned telephone interviews with participants of Phase I to seek feedback on the consultation document titled, *Advancing the Dialogue on Health and Health Care,* and to obtain advice on the implementation of certain options. Using better evidence for better decisions was the main issue presented for further discussion and direction by the Evidence-Based Decision Making Working Group.

Stakeholders conference

Following Phase I consultations, the National Forum on Health sponsored a stakeholders conference, Seeking Solutions to Health and Health Care, in Toronto, April 19-21, 1996. Approximately 200 participants attended, representing health and health care organizations at the national, provincial and community levels. The Evidence-Based Decision Making Working Group chair, Karen Gainer, gave a presentation to plenary at that conference. The theme of the presentation was the Working Group's goals to ensure that decisions about health and health care would be based on the best available evidence at all levels of decision making, including providers, patients, managers and policy makers.

Participants at the conference were assigned to one of 12 workshop groups. Two of the workshop groups discussed opportunities for creating incentives and aligning interests in the system to encourage a culture of evidence-based decision making. The definition of "evidence" was discussed at length, and it was acknowledged that personal judgment and intuition, as well as individual or group priorities and values could influence both the choice and the interpretation of evidence. Finally, the development of the infrastructure to support evidence-based decision making, and the ideal capabilities of Canada's health information infrastructure, were discussed. Stakeholders agreed that there should be a national information infrastructure accessible by consumers/ patients, as well as by providers and policy makers.

Health information dialogue

The Evidence-Based Decision Making Working Group of the National Forum on Health, assembled 10 health information experts from across the country in Vancouver, British Columbia. These experts met with Forum members on May 7 and 8, 1995, to discuss how health information could be used more effectively at provider and policy levels to improve health care practices and decision making. Their presentations contributed in various ways to the Working Group's recommendations on the evaluation of health interventions.

In the field of clinical science, the goal is to ensure that current knowledge is reflected in physician practice. The dialogue focused on

ways to equip policy makers with the tools they require to move research into practice. With respect to population health, participants discussed the information that would be required to ensure that the larger determinants of health, including employment status and social services data would be taken into account by providers and health planners alike. The third general area discussed at the "Dialogue on Health Information" was the health information infrastructure in Canada and investments that should be made in this sector to encourage better resource allocation decisions by managers.

Linkages between key players in the health information sector were expanded by bringing these players together and holding round-table discussions with Forum members. This dialogue contributed knowledge regarding the role of health information in a culture of evidence-based decision making within the Canadian health system.

Consumer dialogue

On June 24 and 25, 1995, the Evidence-Based Decision Making Working Group met with a group of Canadians to discuss levels of satisfaction with available health information and to debate Canadians' current awareness of their health status and the national health system.

Working Group members also had the opportunity to hear the expertise of professionals in various fields. Panellists represented academia, the private health sector, the media, non-profit organizations and health care advocacy groups. Each representative presented her/his perspective on disseminating existing information and generating research results in innovative and accessible ways.

The discussion was organized around three panels, each moderated by consumer participants offering insight from personal experience as decision makers and patients in the formal health care system. The dialogue opened with a discussion of social marketing in the health sector and proceeded to more traditional means of transferring research information to patients. Finally, media representatives and the chair of the Health Council of the Consumers' Association of Canada discussed the types of information that consumers seek on health and health care, as well as the range of options in the popular media permitting public access to this type of information.

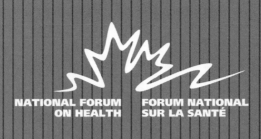

The Need for an Aboriginal Health Institute in Canada

Contents

Introduction 3

The Situation of Aboriginal Peoples. 4

Role of an Aboriginal Health Institute. 7

Development of Human Resources 8

Research and Information – The Foundation for Change 9

Models for Success 10

Conclusion 11

References 12

Introduction

Throughout the multitude of studies, surveys and consultations that have been conducted on, with and about Aboriginal peoples, the message has been consistent: Aboriginal peoples in Canada do not have the same living standards as the rest of the Canadian population, be it educational attainment, housing conditions or income. This is significant given that these are key factors which determine overall health. A critical action in confronting these inequalities relies on finding, developing and using the appropriate information. Recognizing that addressing Aboriginal health inequities requires a multidisciplinary approach, the National Forum on Health is making a number of statements on directions aimed to build the health of Aboriginal peoples (see Determinants of Health and Evidence-Based Decision Making synthesis reports).

In addition to these directions, and based on our research and discussions with Aboriginal peoples, the National Forum on Health proposes the establishment of an Aboriginal health institute. The Forum believes that an institute that would specifically address issues that affect the health of all Aboriginal peoples, would be an important mechanism to bring the full picture of these issues to the surface and advocate for change. The institute would focus on Aboriginal health issues, serve as a support network for Aboriginal health workers in communities, perform and advocate an evidence-based approach in health research to meet the needs of Aboriginal peoples through improved health information. Additionally, the institute would perhaps, most importantly, assist in the sharing of information within and outside of Aboriginal communities.

The Situation of Aboriginal Peoples

We must first recognize that the term Aboriginal peoples does not imply or refer to one homogeneous group. Description of the Aboriginal population is divided into four categories — North American (First Nations) Indians registered under the *Indian Act* (Registered Indians); North American Indians not registered under the *Indian Act*; Métis people; and Inuit (Royal Commission on Aboriginal Peoples, 1996). Each group possesses cultural, linguistic and sometimes geographical distinctions that must be considered when assessing individual health needs.

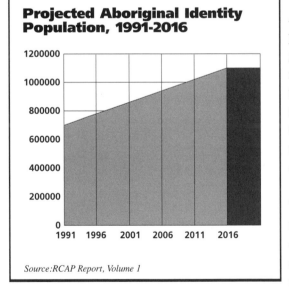

Projected Aboriginal Identity Population, 1991-2016

Source:RCAP Report, Volume 1

The population of Aboriginal peoples in Canada is growing at a more rapid pace than that of the non-Aboriginal Canadian population as the graph demonstrates.

This growth in the population comes as a result of the combination of decreasing infant mortality rates and the higher fertility rates of Aboriginal peoples. This combination also accounts for the "youth" of the Aboriginal population as a whole. As the trend of high fertility and low infant mortality has continued, it is estimated that 38 percent of the Aboriginal population is under the age of 15 as compared to 21 percent in the non-Aboriginal population (CICH, 1994).

Research and appropriate information are needed to understand how the health of Aboriginal peoples are affected by the many risks they face in their daily living. Research commissioned by the Forum concluded that at a broad level, the hardships experienced by Aboriginal peoples are similar to those experienced by all Canadians in similar circumstances. Risk of inadequate income, dependency on welfare, substandard living conditions, stresses on mental health and well-being, physical violence, sexual abuse, and substance abuse are just some of the common factors that threaten the health of Aboriginal peoples. When they occur in combination, these threats to health status are amplified in some Aboriginal populations, with the following results on health, as illustrated in the report of the Royal Commission on Aboriginal Peoples (RCAP) (1996):

■ The life expectancy of Registered Indians[1] is seven to eight years shorter than for non-Aboriginal Canadians.

■ Unemployment rates, incidence of low educational attainment and welfare dependency are higher in First Nations communities.

■ The incidence of violence, physical and sexual abuse and suicide is higher in Aboriginal communities.

[1] *Among Aboriginal peoples, this statistic is available only for Registered Indians.*

- Aboriginal people are increasingly affected by conditions such as cancer and heart disease.

- Children in Aboriginal communities have higher rates of accidental death and injury of all Canadian children.

- Many Aboriginal communities have higher rates of infectious diseases, such as tuberculosis and AIDS than non-Aboriginal Canadians.

There are also risks associated with the socio-economic environment because of unhealthy living conditions such as overcrowded housing with inefficient heating and inadequate water supplies. In addition, Aboriginal peoples have endured the degradation of traditional lands, and its subsequent harmful effects on the environment. This situation has forced a shift away from a subsistence economy where Aboriginal peoples were self-sufficient, to a cash-based economy that increases dependence on government. Unfortunately, many non-Aboriginal Canadians are unaware of or refuse to acknowledge these disparities that damage health. However, in many Aboriginal communities, the situation is, and has been for a long time, at a crisis level.

Although there are a number of issues of concern in Aboriginal communities, the two issues of health status of children and the pandemic of diabetes stand out in their effect on the Aboriginal community, and beg immediacy in dealing with these issues.

There is no doubt that the plight of all Aboriginal peoples is felt most harshly by children. Aboriginal children aged 15 and younger represent only six percent of the total of all Canadian children (CICH, 1994), yet are over-represented in a number of negative health measures. For instance, while it is true that the infant mortality rate among Aboriginal peoples has declined significantly in the past few decades for First Nations peoples, the rate is still double that of the non-Aboriginal population at 14 per 1 000 live births for First Nations peoples versus 7 per 1 000 live births in the non-Aboriginal population (RCAP Report, 1996). Death rates for Indian infants from injuries are four times the rate of non-Aboriginal infants and death rates from other causes such as birth defects, low birth weight, and respiratory illness are consistently and significantly higher among Aboriginal infants and children when compared to the non-Aboriginal population (CICH, 1994).

Aboriginal children are living and growing in conditions that have and will continue to negatively impact health. It has been estimated that 50 percent of Aboriginal children (on or off reserve) are living in poverty and as poor children, they are more likely to have chronic health problems (such as the ones outlined above) as well as psychiatric and emotional disorders (RCAP Report, 1996). The negative risks to the health of all Aboriginal peoples noted earlier are then particularly acute for children. More Aboriginal children than children in the non-Aboriginal population face physical and sexual abuse, face barriers to achieving an adequate level of education, fall victim to substance abuse and commit suicide. In the case of suicide, the Canadian Institute for Child Health reports that between 1986 and 1990, the suicide rate for Indian children 10 to 19 years of age was more than five times the rate of non-Indian children (CICH, 1994). Without question, the state of health for Aboriginal children must become a high priority.

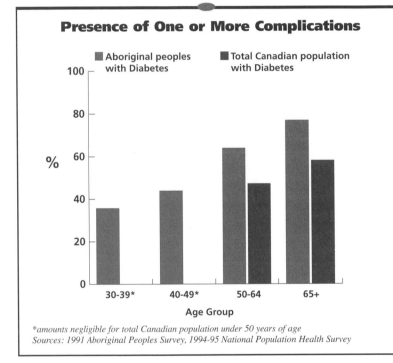

Presence of One or More Complications

■ Aboriginal peoples with Diabetes ■ Total Canadian population with Diabetes

amounts negligible for total Canadian population under 50 years of age
Sources: 1991 Aboriginal Peoples Survey, 1994-95 National Population Health Survey

Of equal concern is the growing pandemic of diabetes among Aboriginal peoples. The evidence available suggests that diabetes disproportionately affects all Aboriginal peoples with the incidence rate, conservatively estimated, being two to three times higher among all Aboriginal than all non-Aboriginal peoples (RCAP Report, 1996). Rates of the disease also vary from region to region and among different Aboriginal groups. What is particularly disturbing is the fact that because symptoms of diabetes develop slowly, they go unrecognized and are diagnosed late in the

development of the disease. It has been estimated that for every known case of diabetes, *at least* one goes undiagnosed (RCAP Report, 1996).

Evidence also suggests that complications from diabetes have been more severe in Aboriginal populations. As the data from the Aboriginal People's Survey conducted in 1991 demonstrates, not only do more First Nations peoples suffer from one or more complications (noted in the survey as high blood pressure, heart disease, and vision problems), but the onset of these complications affects First Nations peoples at an earlier age.

It should be noted that the complications outlined in the survey, do not represent the full extent of the effects of the disease. As well as leading to premature death, diabetes causes medical complications and disability, including kidney disease, heart and circulatory disease, blindness, amputations, nervous system disease, and birth defects among infants born to diabetic mothers (RCAP Report, 1996). It should also be noted that Aboriginal children are being severely affected by this pandemic. More Aboriginal children and youth are developing type II diabetes, also known as late onset diabetes as it most commonly afflicts older persons. Therefore, the evidence suggests that the onset of diabetes in Aboriginal populations occurs at a younger age, is more intensive, and its complications, more severe.

Major risk factors for diabetes include obesity, poor eating habits and physical inactivity. These factors are prevalent in the Aboriginal population primarily as a result of the lifestyle transition that has been imposed on Aboriginal peoples. As Aboriginal peoples have been forced to abandon the traditional subsistence lifestyle that kept people healthy through quality country foods and physical activity through hunting, levels of physical activity have declined, and traditional foods (as well as traditional food preparation methods) have disappeared. The diets of many Aboriginal peoples consist of processed foods with high levels of fat and sugar, that in every way contribute to the ill health, and more specifically to the high incidence of diabetes among all Aboriginal peoples. Recognizing this, increased information, and providing Aboriginal peoples with alternatives to address these issues can play a significant role in reducing the incidence of this disease.

Role of an Aboriginal Health Institute

During the consultations, the Forum heard many participants support and encourage the establishment of an Aboriginal health institute to improve the health of Aboriginal populations. Such an institute, which would be as independent as possible of the political stream of Aboriginal life, would help to identify priorities for health in Aboriginal communities — priorities that would be sensitive to the health and healing needs of Aboriginal peoples and would allow Aboriginal peoples to exercise their own judgement to take control of their health.

It is premature to formulate governance models for the institute without further consultation and direction from Aboriginal peoples. However, the Forum proposes that the institute:

■ be established for, and encourage the participation and contribution of *all* Aboriginal groups;

■ have links with Aboriginal and non-Aboriginal universities and professional organizations. As noted by the RCAP report (1996), "mainstream" institutions can help develop an Aboriginal health institute by offering training opportunities, mentoring and support for new staff, back-up and specialist services, and access to specialized equipment and resources. Additionally, the institute could undertake initiatives to increase admission of Aboriginal students into health professions;

- play a strong advocacy role for Aboriginal peoples. This role becomes especially important in creating linkages with non-Aboriginal organizations and associations;

- aim to replace some of the traditional functions of the Medical Services Branch of Health Canada. That is, the institute would not only support health services at regional and community levels, but would also work with Health Canada (and other government departments including Human Resources Development Canada and Indian and Northern Affairs Canada) to develop different funding initiatives that the institute could access, and form links to a broad range of institutions and networks (such as those for health, the environment and human resources planning); and

- provide the information and direction for addressing diseases such as diabetes. It is long recognized that the lifestyle changes necessary to prevent or control diabetes are different for different groups, however, common to all Aboriginal peoples is the fact that diet and weight control are approached from the point of view of culture, values and experience (RCAP Report, 1996). Hence, culturally relevant and culturally supportive approaches to the management of diabetes, and other chronic and infectious diseases that affect Aboriginal peoples should be developed and implemented both within and outside of Aboriginal communities.

Development of Human Resources

One function of the institute would be training and supporting the education of Aboriginal peoples as health professionals. For Aboriginal peoples to take control of their health and health services, they must become involved in the design, development, delivery and evaluation of services in their communities. This can be facilitated by increasing the number of Aboriginal health professionals. At present, there are approximately 50 Aboriginal physicians; this number represents about 0.1 percent of all physicians in Canada. There are also about 300 Aboriginal registered nurses, again representing about 0.1 percent of the all Canadian nurses (RCAP, Highlights Report 1996). Examples of other health workers in Aboriginal communities include mental health practitioners, nutritionists and dieticians, dental therapists, community health representatives and health administrators. Traditional healers also constitute an important group of Aboriginal health practitioners. Some communities also have services such as alcohol and drug addiction centres.

Encouraging this Aboriginal "strength in numbers" in the health professions will provide a variety of benefits including:

- ensuring that health practices are sensitive to the needs of Aboriginal peoples;

- combining traditional healing practices with contemporary approaches both in and outside of Aboriginal communities;

- providing role models and mentors; and

- through the combination of these benefits, creating best health and better health outcomes for all members of the Aboriginal community.

Research and Information — The Foundation for Change

The creation of an Aboriginal health institute would help to create a solid foundation for research on the health of Aboriginal peoples. It is a widely held view that agendas for Aboriginal research are more often driven by outside interests, not by Aboriginal interests. As a result, initiatives that were supposed to find solutions are inappropriate and may do more harm to communities than good. Aboriginal peoples themselves are often not privy to the results and analysis of the research, robbing communities of the opportunity to learn from, and act on the research. Research must be strengthened in, for example, models for participatory research and survey design. The institute would then facilitate and improve research processes in the Aboriginal context. Improved research results in better information.

For Aboriginal peoples, other than Registered Indians on reserve, there is currently no systematic collection and compilation of person-specific health and health-service utilization data. Medical Services Branch of Health Canada maintains health data, but only for Registered Indians — and advises that "the completeness and quality of the information" is questionable and the data should be "interpreted with caution" (Health Canada, 1996). This means that reliable, comprehensive information regarding all Aboriginal groups is nonexistent, and what information is available cannot be fully trusted.

The institute's wide mandate is needed to fill this information gap in Aboriginal health. Information is required that compares health status, use of health services, and the results of interventions both within Aboriginal communities and with the non-Aboriginal population. Additionally, a critical function of the institute would be to develop an Aboriginal health information infrastructure that:

■ makes reliable information accessible;

■ makes evidence a central element in decision making;

■ employs a multidisciplinary approach in the assessment of the data; and

■ perhaps most importantly, is user friendly at all levels.

Dissemination of this information is also critical. The ideal of an Aboriginal health information system differs in no way from the type of health information system the Forum is proposing for the country as a whole (see Evidence-Based Decison Making working group synthesis report). The system would be comprehensive and rigorous in its research, evaluation and dissemination functions, and would also work to promote accountability.

Models for Success

There are a number of models on which an Aboriginal health institute can be built. One is the concept of the "centre of excellence" which is often characterized by strong links to the private sector and partnerships with government-sponsored health research agencies (e.g., the National Health Research Development Program), universities and professional associations. Provided that both Aboriginal groups and mainstream organizations buy into the concept, these links and partnerships would provide the key for the effectiveness of the proposed Aboriginal health institute. Whether or not the proposed institute would adopt the processes of centres of excellence, such as the competitive aspect of requests for proposals or the degree to which criteria must be satisfied, would be left for future consideration.

Another model is the Centre for Nutrition and the Environment for Indigenous Peoples (CINE). CINE was created, in affiliation with McGill's School of Dietetics and Human Nutrition and the Faculty of Agricultural and Environmental Sciences, to respond to a need expressed by Aboriginal peoples for participatory research and education to address their concerns about the integrity of their traditional food systems. CINE is a permanent research and education resource for and including Aboriginal peoples. The governing board of the centre has representation from the Dene Nation, the Métis, the Inuit and the Assembly of First Nations. This initiative was funded by a private contribution to McGill University specifically for this project and by the Arctic

Environmental Strategy of Canada's Green Plan through Indian and Northern Affairs Canada.

The Saskatchewan Indian Federated College is a model of education and professional training for Aboriginal peoples. In affiliation with the University of Saskatchewan Faculty of Dentistry, the college trains dental therapists to provide services in remote areas in all provinces and territories (except Quebec and Ontario), where dental services have been unavailable. Dental therapist training takes two years. The program is designed to train students to provide basic oral health care services, including fillings, extractions, preventive care and health promotion for children and adults in Aboriginal communities. The program, funded by Health Canada through a five-year contract with the college, operates with an advisory board comprising First Nations peoples, Inuit and a representative of the Canadian Dental Therapists Association. At present, there are 54 dental therapists employed by Health Canada; 24 employed by the Government of the Northwest Territories; 5 employed by the Saskatchewan Northern Health Services Program; and 5 employed by the college. Of these, approximately 30 percent are of Aboriginal ancestry (Health Canada, 1996).

Although these models are somewhat uni-disciplinary and geographically focused, they provide good examples of the kinds of initiatives that are working to improve health for Aboriginal peoples.

Conclusion

In response to what was heard in discussions and in consultations, the National Forum on Health supports and encourages immediate and long term investments to improve the health of Aboriginal peoples. The causes of ill health for Aboriginal peoples, including sub-standard physical environments, the prevalence of chronic and infectious diseases, ssubstance abuse and poverty, must be addressed and effective solutions developed. The establishment of a research-based institute that is controlled by and administered for the benefit of all Aboriginal peoples would play a key role in this effort. The institute must have an advocacy role, base research priorities on needs identified by communities, and incorporate traditional, culturally relevant methods to produce effective solutions. The models for success show that the infrastructure can be put in place for such an initiative, and that Aboriginal communities have successful examples on which to build.

In terms of funding, the Forum believes refocusing Health Canada's current expenditures would mean that little, if any "new" money from government would be needed to establish this institute. There could be opportunities to build more formalized partnerships with private funders who understand the need for Aboriginal peoples to improve their health by being given the opportunity to take control of their health through training, education and information. The CINE example demonstrates that private funders are willing to fund Aboriginal research, and grounding such endeavours in an academic environment may help recruit like-minded funders. This is the challenge, but one that is not impossible.

References

Canada. Health Canada. *Health Programs Analysis, First Nations and Inuit Health Programs*. Ottawa: Indian Health Information Library, 1996.

Canadian Institute for Child Health. *The Health of Canada's Children: A CICH Profile*. Second Edition. Ottawa, 1994.

Royal Commission on Aboriginal Peoples. *Looking Forward, Looking Back — Report of the Royal Commission on Aboriginal Peoples*, Volume 1. Ottawa: Supply and Services Canada, 1996.

_____ . *Gathering Strength – Report of the Royal Commission on Aboriginal Peoples*, Volume 3. Ottawa: Supply and Services Canada, 1996.

_____ . *People to People, Nation to Nation: Highlights from the Report of the Royal Commission on Aboriginal Peoples*. Ottawa: Supply and Services Canada, 1996.

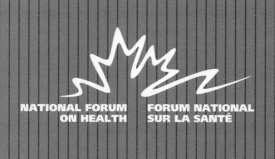

NATIONAL FORUM
ON HEALTH

FORUM NATIONAL
SUR LA SANTÉ

Directions for a Pharmaceutical Policy in Canada

A Joint Report by the Striking a Balance and Evidence–Based Decision Making Working Groups

Striking a Balance Working Group

Steven Lewis (Chair)
William R.C. Blundell, B.A.Sc.
Richard Cashin, LL.B.
André–Pierre Contandriopoulos, Ph.D.
Robert G. Evans, Ph.D.
Tom W. Noseworthy, M.D.

Evidence–Based Working Group

Karen Gainer LL.B. (Chair)
Mamoru Watanabe, M.D. (Chair)
Robert G. Evans, Ph.D.
Margaret McDonald, R.N.
Eric M. Maldoff, LL.B.
Tom W. Noseworthy, M.D.
Noralou P. Roos, Ph.D.
Lynn Smith, LL.B., Q.C.

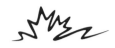

Contents

Background 3

Pharmaceuticals and the Health Care System 10

Goals for Pharmaceutical Reform 11

Pharmaceutical Reform: Key Elements 13

    Access Through Public Management 13

    Information as the Key to Management 13

    Integration of Services 14

    Management of Costs 15

    Funding Pharmaceuticals 17

Recommendations 18

Endnotes 20

References 21

Background

Between 1975 and 1994 Canadian expenditures on drugs increased from $1.1 to $9.2 billion. Expenditures per person, adjusted for inflation, more than doubled, rising from $108 to $232. Drug expenditures increased faster than any other major category of health care; their share of total health spending thus rose from 8.7 percent to 12.7 percent.[1] Prescription drugs made up about seventy percent of this total, $6.5 billion in 1994, the remainder being non-prescription or over-the-counter (OTC) drugs and personal health supplies.

Drugs are financed from a combination of public and private sources, but private funding accounts for a much larger share — about two-thirds of the total — than it does of hospital and physician costs. OTC drugs and supplies are entirely privately funded, while the public sector pays for less than half — just over forty-five percent — of prescription drugs. This represents a significant increase since 1975, however, when the public share of prescription drug costs was only twenty percent.

No province has a universal drug plan providing first dollar coverage to all residents. Most provide prescription drugs for seniors (in one case only for those receiving the Guaranteed Income Supplement) and for welfare recipients. Three provinces (British Columbia, Saskatchewan, Manitoba) provide some coverage to all residents, with substantial individual "contributions" (user charges) in the form of co-payments and/or deductibles. (The former require the patient to pay either a percentage of the total bill or a fixed amount per bill; the latter limit coverage to charges beyond a certain level per person or family in a given time period.) Quebec is about to institute a universal drug plan with similar features.

The Canadian Pharmaceutical Association reports that public plans cover about 44 percent of Canadians. Private plans are provided for or purchased by another 44 percent (see also CROP Conseil, 1995), while 12 percent are without any drug insurance coverage and must pay out of pocket the full charge for each prescription drug required. OTC drugs are, as noted, not included in public insurance. Since both public and private insurance plans typically require beneficiaries to pay part of the cost of insured drugs out-of-pocket, however, the proportion of people covered does not correspond to the proportion of total costs reimbursed. In fact, deductible amounts in provinces with "universal" plans covering all residents are set sufficiently high that relatively few residents will actually receive any reimbursement.

The total payment for drug benefits by private insurers in 1993 is estimated at $2.2 billion (CROP Conseil, 1995), or about 65% of the total private expenditures on prescription reported by Health Canada for that year. This would imply that out of pocket expenses amount to about 20% [0.35x0.55] of total outlays. But total private drug benefits include reimbursement for certain forms of non–prescription drugs as well. In so far as $2.2 billion overstates the amount of private reimbursement for prescription drugs alone, the 20% estimate above correspondingly understates the proportion paid for out-of-pocket.

Private coverage is often included in employment benefit packages, with partial or full premium payment by the employer; this has tax advantages because the employee is not taxed on this benefit as s/he would be on a corresponding amount in wages.[2] Accordingly people with private drug insurance tend to be in full–time, stable employment in "good" jobs with generous benefit packages — and are correspondingly relatively healthy. Such jobs are also, on average, better paid. People whose attachment to the labour force is, for whatever reason, partial, unstable, or non-existent, are much less likely to have access to private coverage — or to be able to afford it if they did.[3]

The result is that private drug insurance is correlated with income, not with need. A survey in 1995 (CROP Conseil, 1995) found that 75% of Canadians earning more than $60,000 a year had private insurance, dropping to 68% in the range $40–$60,000, 42% in the $20–$40,000 range and 7% below $20,000. Partly as a result, per capita out of pocket drug expenses of higher income households are on average lower than those of lower income households, and much lower as a share of income (Lexchin, 1996).

The cost of private plans has nonetheless been growing, prompting large companies to seek ways to limit their expenses. Private plans have generally been less restrictive than public plans in delineating what drugs are covered, but are attempting to become more so. Alternatively, employers are considering flexible benefit programs. The employer provides a fixed dollar amount toward the cost of benefits, offers a host of plans with varying degrees of coverage, and the employee selects among plans on the basis of the preferred package of services, and his/her willingness to make a contribution beyond what is provided by the employer. In general, employer-sponsored plans have responded to rising costs by trying to limit the plan's exposure, and shift costs onto beneficiaries, rather than trying to manage overall costs.

Studies indicate that drugs are both over–utilized and inappropriately used (Coambes et al., 1995; Tamblyn and Perrault, 1997). Such concerns have a long history; their persistence indicates the absence of any significant incentive for response. Inappropriate use includes taking drugs in the wrong dosage, at the wrong time, not long enough, not at all, or in combination with other drugs or substances. This can occur as a result of either inappropriate prescribing or failure of the patient to comply with the prescription (or both). The latter may be a consequence of lack of information, or inadvertence, or carelessness. It may also be traceable to the nature of the clinical contact — what did the physician say and the patient hear? Inappropriate prescribing, on the other hand, raises questions about the behaviour of clinicians and pharmaceutical manufacturers and the incentives, including economic motivations, to which they respond. It is a much more sensitive subject than non-compliance, which leads only to questions about how to improve *patient* behaviour.

Over-prescribing is the result of complex factors involving patients, physicians and manufacturers. At root, however, the forces at work are very simple. The cost structure of the pharmaceutical industry creates very powerful economic incentives forcing manufacturers constantly to expand their sales. Massive resources are thus put into highly sophisticated marketing campaigns; and successful marketing means more drugs sold — more utilization. At the same time, the pressures of fee-for-service medical practice make the prescription a critical stage in closing off a patient visit, symbolizing that the problem has been understood and the therapy chosen. Physician incomes are directly linked to the rate at which patients are moved through the office, and heavy prescribing is linked with a high throughput practice style (Davidson *et al.* 1994). One should not, therefore, be surprised to see a steady rise in drug expenditures; these are the rising sales of a successful industry, meeting the needs of practitioners.

On the other hand Coambes et al. in a comprehensive review on behalf of the Pharmaceutical Manufacturers Association of Canada, focus attention on non-compliance by patients. They estimate that the direct (patients seeking additional medical therapy), and indirect costs (loss of productivity) resulting from non-compliance with therapies for major chronic diseases in Canada, amounted to $7 to $9 billion per year; figures labelled as a "conservative estimate." (Coambes et al., 1995). These "indirect costs" are, however, estimates of potential losses of output elsewhere in the economy; they do not show up as part of total health care expenditures.

The Canadian public is very concerned about drug costs and over-utilization of drugs. Access limitations, on the other hand, are less visible to the public. During nation-wide discussion groups, participants expressed the view that physicians and drug companies form a unholy alliance which they blame for high demand, and consequent high usage of pharmaceuticals. They are also sceptical of the economic benefits alleged to flow from the

adoption of Bill C-91,[4] which in 1993 eliminated compulsory licensing.[5] They recognize that its intended effect, as with any patent legislation, is to limit competition and raise prices and industry profits, thus contributing to the overall escalation of health care costs in Canada. But they find less plausible the argument that these costs will be off-set, at some later date, by increased availability of new and more effective drugs that will improve health outcomes and perhaps lower care costs. New drugs will undoubtedly become available, but the causal link to Bill C-91 is a separate issue.

The dynamics of the pharmaceutical sector are such that the players are in fierce competition with one another to establish brand-name recognition of their products by physicians, to build consumer allegiance, and to garner profits from the sale of these products.[6] After reflection upon the sums of money spent on advertising and the extent of detailing (informational visits to physicians) by company sales representatives, we have concluded that these activities to promote products and increase sales do not always reflect what is in the patient's best interest. Many doctors have neither the time nor the familiarity with pharmaceuticals to compare and contrast information they receive from manufacturers. If salesmen could be expected to provide objective information on alternative drug and healing interventions, their interaction with doctors could be most beneficial. But such an expectation would be naive. A salesman's job is to sell, and only to sell; that is what s/he is paid for. Providing objective information may in some circumstances be one means to this end, but is not in general. Nor are salesmen paid to promote competitors' products. Studies have shown that even print advertisements exaggerate clinical benefits of advertised drugs (Lexchin, 1994; Wivell and O'Fallon, 1992).

Some advocate direct advertising to consumers, on the argument that this will reduce the asymmetry of information between patient and provider. The patient might then have more influence in what is otherwise perceived as a profit-making alliance between providers and manufacturers. The asymmetry of information, however, is why marketing of pharmaceutical products is regulated in the first place. The subject is highly technical, and the industry, transnational. Monitoring prices, quality and efficacy requires comparison of clinical trials, scientific research incentives and comparative governmental regulation. The notion that advertisers would choose to act as educators trying to remedy patients' lack of information, rather than as marketers trying to exploit it, seems to lack any obvious motivation. It is inconsistent with the economic incentives involved, and is not supported by any evidence.

Nonetheless, drugs have a greater similarity to a 'consumer product' than do most other medical services. Over-the-counter drugs in particular are widely available and easily accessible on drug store shelves or in other retail stores. For many conditions it may be possible to choose between OTC and prescription drugs, and even when there is no OTC alternative, there will often be a choice between generic and brand name versions of the same drug, or among different but therapeutically equivalent drugs. In principle, and often in practice, it may be possible for patients to acquire the information necessary to make a rational choice. But the investment of time and energy, and the intellectual demands, may be considerable. To have thousands of consumers actively researching drug therapies and confronting personal physicians with alternatives, seems like at best an inefficient way to improve the quality of prescribing, and at worst totally implausible.

The Working Groups on Striking a Balance and Evidence-Based Decision Making have concluded that reasonable restrictions on pharmaceutical marketing practices are justified. In particular, professional licensing authorities and educational institutions should take a stronger stand to shield students in the health professions from drug company representatives, and to limit the use of sponsorships and subsidies to professionals. Making those practices more visible to the general public may help to place limits on their use. Similarly, direct-to-consumer advertising for prescription drugs should not be allowed; current legislative loopholes should be closed. Finally, careful scrutiny should be given to the practice of shifting prescription drugs to OTC status. Manufacturers of brand name products seek approval for OTC sale to extend a product's profitable life after the expiry of patent protection. Once a product is approved for OTC sale, the manufacturer may effectively block generic competition through massive expenditures on marketing; the low prices of generic drugs are based on almost non-existent marketing costs (Morgan, 1997). Presently, this shift is limited to drugs for easily self-diagnosed conditions which do not require additional clinical management. Over-the-counter status should not be given to other types of pharmaceuticals.

Government regulation of the drug industry meets with widespread public acceptance. Governments approve the safety of drugs, license the purveyors and regulate prices. But governments also regulate on behalf of the industry, or at least certain of its member firms, to create favourable investment opportunities by establishing and upholding intellectual property rights on new discoveries. The justification offered for the resulting restrictions on competition and increases in prices is that pharmaceutical companies will invest some of their increased profits in supporting both in-house and extra-mural (university-based) research. An industry promise to increase support for research was an explicit *quid pro quo* for the benefits they recieved from Bill C-91.

The Forum's role, in part, was to investigate the overall arrangement between governments, manufacturers, professionals, and the public. We found that governments are not doing enough to inform consumers, provide access to essential pharmaceuticals, control prescription and non-prescription drug expenditures, and encourage research on new chemical products. As we stated earlier, twelve percent of Canadians have no insurance coverage for drugs, while out-of-pocket payments amount to twenty percent or more of costs of prescription drugs, as well as nearly all non-prescription drugs and related supplies. Prices of new drugs are still considered by a number of experts to be high.[7]

Finally, public investment in, and promotion of, research by multinational firms, does not necessarily provide the greatest return for Canadians. Research efforts in Canada focus on two areas: variations of existing drugs that provide moderate or no therapeutic improvement over existing medicines ("me-too" drugs); and line extensions (usually a new strength) of existing medicines. The alternative of course, is to do more basic research—work that advances scientific knowledge without a specific application in view. In 1995, basic research accounted for only 22.2 percent of current R&D expenditures (PMPRB, 1996).

An unlooked for consequence of Bill C–91, and the corresponding industry commitment to increased research funding, is that the drug industry has now become a predominant source of funding for biomedical research in Canada. Public sources, both federal and provincial, have been much more restricted. But at the end of the day the industry's research efforts and priorities are ultimately driven by the prospects for development of profitable products and favourable marketing environments. That is, after all, the fiduciary duty of management to the shareholders. Consequently there is the potential, indeed the virtual certainty, that the whole direction of biomedical research, and of health research more generally, will be narrowed in focus and skewed in the direction of drug– and product–related research. Research to improve our understanding of the determinants of health, or the management of health care services, have no payoff to drug industry shareholders.

At the same time researchers, and their sponsoring institutions, become hostage to the political priorities of the industry. They must become advocates and lobbyists for the drug industry, in order to ensure the survival of their own research programs. Yet the research funding that the industry distributes is ultimately derived from the Canadian public through the higher prices made possible by increased patent protection.

The only way to mitigate the "steering" effect of expanded industry support for research is to move the administration and allocation of those research funds away from the control of the industry itself, and into the hands of the public granting agencies.[8] It is important to emphasize that it is the steering effect, the channelling of such a major share of Canadian research talent and funding into a very narrow and commercially focused range of questions, that is the problem, not the quality or integrity of the review process or the research itself. "Partnerships" between the industry and particular granting agencies do not help; their research focus is still on drugs. The transfer must be arm's length, with no strings.

Nor is our concern only with externally supported research. The drug industry's commitment to carry out more of its internal research in Canada is also underwritten by the increase in Canadian-source revenues that it derives from Bill C-91. The funding that the pharmaceutical industry contributes to public granting agencies, to be allocated on the basis of national research priorities, not simply for more drugs, should include *all* the additional research support, in-house as well as extramural, that was to have been "purchased" by Canadians through the privileges conferred by Bill C-91.

Participants in the National Stakeholder Conference, held in April 1996, felt that pharmaceutical policy needed adjustment on a range of issues including: over-utilization, physician prescribing practices, direct marketing to physicians, lack of effective information systems, the role of drugs in the health care system, perverse incentives in the fee-for-service reimbursement system including compensating the pharmacist for each prescription written, consumer behaviour, alternative therapies and drug safety. The surging cost of prescription and non-prescription drugs was noted, and Bill C-91 was cited as a source of high prices. Forum members also heard requests for government to play an increasing role in determining the focus of research activities. Finally, stakeholders expressed concerns about the limitations of the Patented Medicine Prices Review Board's mandate.[9]

Against this backdrop, it is of particular interest to note several recently instituted changes in provincial drug benefit programs that have put issues of access and cost of drugs on the front pages.

Ontario started charging a co-payment for welfare recipients and people over 65 in an attempt to recoup the burden of costs in the public system. In effect the province has chosen not to address overall drug costs, but to reduce pressure on public budgets by shifting costs to users. Apart from any concerns that this approach might raise about access by people with very limited resources, past experience suggests that the effects will be one-time only and that the escalation of overall — and of public — costs will continue.

Quebec announced a plan to make prescription drug coverage universal, supported by revenues from general taxes, premiums and co-payments. While the Quebec plan represents a new benefit for many employed adults, it is seen as a reduction of benefits (or an increase in contributions) for welfare recipients and seniors. It was not meant to replace private plans but rather to fill in the gaps between existing public and private plans.[10] Although "universal", the Quebec plan does not have a single source of payment. The mix of public and private insurers, combined with continued private payment, has been shown to make cost control, let alone more effective system management, difficult or impossible in other sectors of health care.

British Columbia already has a nominally "universal" drug program, although for the under 65 population the deductibles are (deliberately) set high enough that there are few beneficiaries, and the coverage for those over 65, which was once first-dollar, now includes a co-payment (whose introduction did not stem the increase in costs). The new element is a system known as "reference-based pricing" under which drugs that may be quite different in their chemical composition and mode of action, but that are used to respond to the same clinical problem — the various forms of ulcer therapy, for example — are assigned to the same reference class. If the research literature indicates these different drugs are equally effective, then the provincial plan will pay only for the lowest cost drug in each reference class. (Physicians may, on application, have an exception made for any individual patient.) The resulting system functions like an ideal, fully informed market, reducing the sales of products whose higher price is not matched by increased value. It is a logical extension of policies to encourage the substitution of lower-cost generic drugs for high-priced branded equivalents, policies that will become less effective as Bill C–91 reduces the availability of generic substitutes.

Of these three policy changes, only the B.C. approach is actually aimed at reducing drug costs and improving prescribing appropriateness. Keeping in mind that expenditures on prescription drugs represent the sales revenue of the drug industry (and of pharmacies), it should not be surprising that the industry's response to reference-based pricing has been bitter opposition, and attacks on the political, legal, and economic levels. The Ontario and Quebec approaches have generated no such hostility. Indeed given the balance of economic interests, it is probably not too far-fetched to suggest that the probable effect on drug costs of any public (or private) reimbursement policy can be gauged by the tone and vigour of the industry's response.

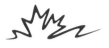

Pharmaceuticals and the Health Care System

Pharmaceuticals have always played an important role in health and health care. They save lives, prevent the spread of disease, help in diagnosis, improve the quality of life for many, and control pain and suffering. Their role is likely to grow in the future as technological advances in pharmacotherapy replace earlier treatment modalities or introduce therapies where none existed before. At the same time advances in other areas (new surgical instruments, new procedures, new anaesthetics, etc.) have changed patterns of health care, particularly in hospitals, resulting in shorter lengths of stay and in substitution of "ambulatory" or same-day treatment, for inpatient care.

Average length of stay in hospitals is decreasing, in part because acute and non-acute services can be provided in less medically and technologically-intensive environments. It is also the case that in the past, inpatient lengths of stay were typically based on historical conventions, arbitrarily arrived at. Increasing pressures on hospital budgets have forced physicians — and nurses — to abandon old habits and discover "new" standards that were, in fact, always possible. But whatever their cause, falling lengths of stay have implications for drug reimbursement.

Our current system provides full funding for acute institutional care, including all drugs provided during a hospital stay. But when a patient is discharged this expense is transferred to the patient, or his/her (public or private) insurer. Yet our goal is, or should be, to rationalize costs — to fund the service or product, not the institution where the care is delivered. There is no logical or equitable reason why drug costs should be transferred from the institution to individuals, as a by-product of the process of making more appropriate use of hospitals. The current situation is not only unfair, it is also inefficient. Hospitals have been able to hold down their drug costs through competitive tendering processes, including volume discounts, and can manage the dispensing process to make best use of hospital pharmacists. Patients at home have no such opportunities for volume purchasing, and face both higher costs of information and minimal opportunities to negotiate prices.

The pace of change in hospitals and concurrent efforts to restructure the provision of health services will likely increase concerns about access and utilization, and continue to put upward pressure on drug costs. Measures taken to date by public and private payers have not brought the growth of pharmaceutical costs in line with that of the rest of the health care system.[11] Most measures have targeted one or the other factor or player but so far, none has appeared to get to the heart of the incentives at play. Furthermore, the multiplicity of players has prevented concerted action. The various opportunities for cost shifting have distracted attention from the much more complex and controversial process of actual management and control.[12]

In considering the options open to government, members of the National Forum on Health have taken into account the success of governments in controlling overall health

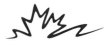

expenditures in the last few years, as well as success stories from abroad. Members believe that a comprehensive approach is needed.

Goals for Pharmaceutical Reform

The reforms proposed here were designed to achieve two principal goals, in light of the intrinsic value of pharmaceuticals in a continuum of care and their increasing importance as a proportion of health care expenditures. First and most obviously, prescription drugs have as good a claim to "medical necessity" as medical and hospital services, implying that access to drugs should be accorded equal importance. Secondly, however, and notwithstanding the private-for-profit, highly competitive environment in which drug development and marketing takes place, the status of drugs as an essential public good makes them prone to cost escalation without limit. Comprehensive controls will be necessary to slow the growth of prescription drug expenditures.

The information acquired from international comparisons of health expenditures, and a collection of papers on pharmaceutical issues, contributed to the development of this view. These included information on the non-medical interventions which influence the health of Canadians, and dealt with the social and psychological conditions which contribute to health or ill-health. Many of these (e.g. depression, suicide, isolation) have come to be medicalized, and treated pharmacologically. In formulating its advice, the Forum took into account the views held by Canadians on health, health care and drugs, as expressed through work commissioned by the Values Working Group, through various phases of the consultation process, and through written submissions.

That drugs are as much a part of "medically necessary" care as are the services of physicians and of hospitals, seems now too obvious to deserve discussion. But this raises an issue that runs deeper than questions of access, appropriateness, and equity. In a fundamental sense, it implies that we do not wish to treat drugs as a "commodity", on a par with shoes and ships and sealing wax, and that it is irrational and inconsistent with our broader objectives to do so.

In the ordinary marketplace, sellers of commodities market their products to anyone who can be persuaded to buy. But "medically necessary" services are of value when, and only when, provided to those who can benefit from them. Providing services to others is not only useless but may be actually harmful. Hospitals and physicians are not expected or professionally encouraged to "market" their services; rather they are expected to meet the needs of patients, and to refrain from providing, indeed to withhold, services that are not appropriate.[13]

Drugs, on the other hand, are marketed with great energy and skill, by firms whose managements are responsible for maximizing their profits. Increasing sales — that is, escalating drug costs — and continuing concerns about over-prescribing are not a "side-effect", but the direct and natural consequence of this behaviour. They are indicators of industry success. At the same time, of course, the considerable expense of this marketing effort has to be included in the price of the drugs themselves and contributes to higher prices.

To a large extent the peculiar difficulties in formulating public policy toward drugs, in

Canada and elsewhere, can be attributed to a profound inconsistency on this issue — are drugs market commodities, or health care services? Consistent application to drugs of the principles that apply in the hospital and physicians' services sectors would imply "de-commodification" of drugs, and in particular active discouragement of drug marketing through both regulatory and purchasing policies. This would lead both to lower prices, and to more appropriate prescribing.

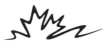

Pharmaceutical Reform: Key Elements

Access Through Public Management

The National Forum on Health believe that the way to improve appropriate access to, and utilization of drugs, and to control the growth of drug expenditures, is to ensure that medically necessary prescription[13] drugs are made available to all Canadian residents, without deductibles or co-payments. International experience has shown that this is best accomplished under a publicly financed and regulated system, which in Canada would, of course, be administered by the provinces with arrangements for portability of benefits — within reasonable constraints — throughout the country. In essence, that requires finding a mechanism to transfer private health expenditures to governments so that they can be managed publicly.[14]

This is the ideal the Forum advocates for the long term. Because financing issues are intrinsically tied to the organization of the health system, and because the organization of our health system is in flux, we can only go so far as to recommend the characteristics of the system that will promote improved management of pharmaceuticals. It will be the responsibility of federal and provincial governments to establish financial and other incentives that will direct and synchronize reforms across the country. Our proposals should be seen as incremental and interdependent: each requiring political will, financial backing, and persuasive leadership. As a first step toward

improving access, we need better information to monitor and evaluate utilization at the individual level, and to facilitate decision making at federal and provincial levels.

Information as the Key to Management

The development within each province of automated, interactive state of the art decision support tools (e.g. disease management information systems) would assist physicians and patients in making appropriate clinical decisions. The potential of the public system to control cost and utilization will not be fully realized without a comprehensive, population-based health information system which allows for a core set of analyses at both provincial and regional authority levels (NFOH, Evidence, 1997).

Specifically, drug monitoring systems should be a priority area for development. These systems would be characterized by central information links between physicians, pharmacists, government paying agencies and the public. As well, they should support reimbursement plans, clinical practice guidelines and utilization review. Ideally, information sources would be developed to respond to questions likely to be posed by the many actors who could benefit from comprehensive information. Consumers might inquire into the side effects of a particular medication, for example, whereas physicians might determine contraindications and interactions with other medications.

At the same time, careful attention must be given to the protection of individual records. Consumers are already wary that medically-related information on individuals, when compiled into databases, might then be sold to pharmaceutical manufacturers, or other interested parties. The privacy and confidentiality of this information must be protected. We need to distinguish between commercial uses of data and uses of data as part of the treatment and research processes. And then we need to encrypt data, authorize users, and pass enforceable legislation that acknowledges that both commercial and public interests are at play (NFOH, Evidence, 1997).

Integration of Services

During the Forum's public consultations, a high degree of consensus was achieved on the need for greater integration of health services. Stakeholders and public participants recommended reforms to the system of primary care, including "one-stop shopping" for all health-related services. In general, services are seen as too compartmentalized. The Forum agrees with this assessment. Links between providers, hospitals, and continuing care services must be strengthened to ensure smooth transitions for patients in the health system.

There have been some attempts across the country at reforming primary care over the past quarter century, including CLSCs (Centres Locaux de Services Communautaires) in Quebec, Health Service Organizations in Ontario, and Community Health Centres in Ontario, Manitoba and Saskatchewan. Outside Quebec, however, these have been on a very small scale. More recent provincial initiatives to integrate the provision of care services at the regional level have been applied across the whole population. But in all cases, funding and decision–

making structures for physician services and drug programs have remained centralized at the provincial level.

The Striking a Balance Synthesis Report recommends that efforts be stepped up across the country to reform primary care with a view to greater integration and coordination of services. Stating that it is premature to come out in favour of any one form of allocation mechanism, the Report states that population-based funding, multidisciplinary teams of providers, and defined geographic or roster-based service populations should be key characteristics of reform (NFOH, Balance, 1997). The report recommends pilot projects which incorporate these features, as well as various ways of remunerating providers. It is within this context of ongoing and proposed initiatives to improve the integration of services, that the Working Groups on Striking a Balance and Evidence-Based Decision Making propose to address pharmaceutical cost and management issues.

Given that similar problems of cost escalation and over-utilization are faced world-wide, it is helpful to look at international examples. In some countries (particularly Germany and the U.K.) drug and physician remuneration budgets have been integrated to make physician incomes or practice revenues partly dependent (negatively) on prescribing volume. Such integration, which recognizes the obvious fact that the prescribing physician is the critical actor in the chain of drug use, have had some success in decreasing drug expenditures[15]. Experiments with that approach, in (or even out of) the context of primary care reform, are worth pursuing.

Instituting a system in which public funding for prescription drugs and for pharmacists' dispensing fees are integrated with budgets for physicians' remuneration, would present challenges on various fronts. Physicians would be challenged to improve the management of pharmaceuticals as a component of their practice. They would likely monitor more closely their patients' utilization of drugs and compliance with prescribed regimens.

This arrangement might also bring community pharmacists into a role similar to that of hospital pharmacists, whose knowledge of pharmacology can in fact be applied in clinical management and utilization review. Drug distribution is already changing with the emergence of mail-order pharmacies and other innovations facilitated by communication technology and modern retailing. Reform of primary care could be the opportunity (as mail order pharmacy may be the stimulus) for pharmacists finally to leave dispensing to technicians, and become more involved in professional services and direct patient care.

These developments are in keeping with increased patient demand for information about health matters and for involvement in decisions concerning their personal health and the management of their care. To permit this shift, governments should review regulations pertaining to dispensing so as to provide patients with a variety of options for obtaining their prescribed drugs. This review could take place under the umbrella of the Conference of Deputy Ministers of Health, with appropriate professional and consumer representation.

Provincial governments are actively discussing alternatives for primary care reform — seen here as an opportunity for pharmaceutical reform. The federal government can be a catalyst in this process by providing a 'transition fund' to provinces to pilot and evaluate health care delivery innovations. The Balance Synthesis Report recommends federal funding to support strategic projects and investments.

Management of Costs

Pharmaceutical policy cannot be addressed in isolation. Drug reimbursement programs must incorporate a number of cost control measures including initiatives proven successful in other industrialized countries. One option is to limit the range of pharmaceutical products eligible for reimbursement. Positive lists specify which drugs will be reimbursed and exclude all others; negative lists exclude specific products and cover all others. Both types of list constitute a formulary; these are increasingly used by governments and private payers both to discourage inappropriate prescribing and to control costs.

While a national formulary for Canada might be considered, it is probably not necessary and could take a long time to develop. Unless provinces began to refuse reimbursement for drugs that were obviously "medically necessary", there would be no reason not to let each province establish its own rules. Based on the experience of the last thirty years with medical care, it is probable that a program with broad national conditions would result in similar formularies across the country (while allowing for some inter–provincial variation). Rhetoric aside, provincial variations in coverage have not been a significant problem with Medicare — at least to date.

Whichever drugs may be covered, however, payers have long been aware of the major differences in prices charged for brand name and generic versions of the same drug. They have over the years introduced a variety of measures to encourage physicians to prescribe and pharmacists to dispense generically. When pursued comprehensively, as Canada did with the compulsory licensure policy between 1969 and the mid-1980s, such approaches can significantly reduce drug costs. As noted above, however, the abandonment of this policy by the federal government will in all likelihood delay and reduce the availability of generic competitor drugs in the future (that being its specific intent) and thus reduce the effectiveness of this form of cost control.

Hence the significance of British Columbia's introduction of reference-based pricing for prescription drugs. It opens up substitution among drugs within a group of medicines interchangeable in terms of clinical effect, even if the drugs themselves differ in chemical composition and mode of action. The provincial government's reimbursement rate is then set equal to the price of the least costly drug in this group. As the potential for generic substitution among exact chemical equivalents is reduced following the abandonment of compulsory licensure and the extension of patent lives, this policy introduces an even wider range of possible substitutions. On the other hand it will be limited in so far as there may not be, for a particular branded drug, *any* other that is interchangeable in clinical effect.

Direct price regulation is a more difficult question; there is room for some differences of opinion as to the effectiveness of the Patented Medicine Prices Review Board (PMPRB) in regulating the price of patented drugs. The Forum believes that the PMPRB can continue to play a useful role, though as noted above the critical stage in drug pricing is at the point of first listing. In any case, given the jurisdictional issues surrounding the regulation of non-patented drugs, and given the absence of any hard evidence pointing to excessive prices in this area, the Forum does not recommend that the Board's mandate be expanded to incorporate non–patented drugs.

On the other hand, there does appear to be good evidence that aggressive drug purchasing, in bulk and if necessary on the international market, can lead to substantial reductions in drug costs. Hospitals in Canada acquire drugs at significantly lower costs than are available to individual patients purchasing through community pharmacies. And Australia, again purchasing aggressively on the world market, appears to be able to supply its people with drugs at a much lower cost than obtains in Canada. Firms in the United States, that specialize in "Pharmaceutical Benefits Management" offer their private-sector clients — typically large employers paying for their employees' drug insurance — substantial savings through aggressive purchasing of both ingredients and dispensing services.[16] There seems to be room for a good deal of experimentation, and study of others' experience, in this area.

Funding Pharmaceuticals

In the current fee-for-service system, physician remuneration could be increased to provide budgets to pay for drugs prescribed out of hospital. In a new primary care environment, ambulatory drugs could be included in capitation funding formulas. These integrated budgets would achieve the dual goals of cost control and making drug use a more integral component of total care.

We are not proposing to increase overall spending ($6.5 billion in 1994) but rather attempting to control its future growth and to improve access. We are recommending full first-dollar coverage (i.e. no user fees) for prescription drugs for all Canadians, however, fiscal reality in the 1990s is such that this will not happen overnight. Over time, we propose to shift private spending on prescribed pharmaceuticals (estimated at $3.6 billion in 1994) to public funding. We believe that this will broaden access, improve equity, and make possible better overall cost control. We would therefore recommend that the federal government undertake with provincial and territorial governments, private payers, consumers and health professionals to explore various organizational models, their funding requirements and implementation strategies.

In the meantime both new and existing measures for achieving cost control, through both regulatory and purchasing policies should be introduced and evaluated. Canadians are very concerned about health in general and pharmaceutical management is one of the areas in which they are most supportive of government involvement. *Most of these initiatives will be taken at the provincial level, and can as the British Columbia example shows be applied to that component of pharmaceutical spending that is already a provincial responsibility.*

Public policy toward drugs is further complicated, in several ways, by the multi-national character of the industry. Not least of the difficulties is the demonstrated ability of the industry to bring international pressure to bear, through foreign governments, to modify Canadian policies in its interest. On the other hand, it may be that concerted action with other countries, initiated by the federal Minister of Health, could be a more effective counterweight to these pressures. Many countries are struggling with exactly the same problems of managing drug utilization and costs.

Canadians should expect to see continuous change and experimentation with integrated models in the coming decade. Public consultations have led the National Forum to recommend public funding for medically necessary services regardless of where they are provided, and by whom (NFOH, Balance, 1997). By and large, these changes should improve the efficiency and quality of health services provided that the system retains its single-payer, publicly-financed character. As we stated earlier, reconciling the profit-driven, private sector ethos of the drug manufacturing industry with the understanding that drugs are an essential public good, will not be easy. Public policy, however, must safeguard what is in the best interests of the public. We believe that our proposals embody the core values that Canadians hold in regard to health and health care.

Recommendations

The Working Groups therefore recommend:

a) That pharmaceutical payment policy in Canada be guided by the goals of:
— equity of access;
— improved prescribing appropriateness; and
— cost–containment;

and that to these ends the Canadian federal-provincial health insurance system move toward integration of prescription drugs as a fully funded component of publicly funded health care.

b) That the reform process begin with the implementation of comprehensive, population-based drug information systems. These must be publicly run databases, capturing all prescription information regardless of payer, such as now exists in Saskatchewan and British Columbia. They can serve to link physicians, pharmacists, patients and provincial payers, and can then support improved clinical decision-making;, utilization review; patient information; and innovations in reimbursement policies such as extensions of bulk purchasing, the British Columbia reference-based pricing system, or developments in "pharmaceutical benefits management systems" in the United States.

c) That the federal government should undertake to support and assist provincial efforts to manage drug utilization and costs, and avoid initiating any policies that might create impediments to such efforts, while at the same time employing similar management approaches in areas where it has direct responsibility for drug reimbursement — e.g. for Status Indians, Veterans, etc.

d) That as provinces develop experiments with integrated primary health care funding envelopes allocated to community-based agencies, budgets for physicians' remuneration be expanded to cover charges for publicly funded prescription drugs (both ingredients and dispensing fees).

e) That current prohibitions against marketing prescription drugs directly to consumers be maintained, and that such marketing continue to be restricted to health professionals, but that in addition schools that educate health professionals follow the lead of McMaster University Medical School, in prohibiting drug marketers from having direct access to students, other than through the director of their program.

f) That during the up-coming mandatory review of Bill C-91 in 1997, the commitments to increased funding for research made by the pharmaceutical industry at the time of its initial passage be converted into specific required contributions to a fund for health research broadly defined, at full arm's length from the industry, to be administered by the national research granting agencies and allocated through the normal peer-reviewed granting process.

g) That while domestic measures to manage drug utilization, improve effectiveness, and control costs are pursued with vigour wherever possible; efforts should also be made to initiate concerted action at the international level.

h) That the federal government, provincial governments, health care providers, private payers (employers, unions and the public) should begin discussions immediately to develop a plan to integrate prescription drugs as a component of publicly funded and administered health care as fiscal resources and management technology permit.

Endnotes

1 *National Health Expenditures in Canada, 1975–1994*, January 1996, Part 3, page 11. These data represent expenditures on prescribed drugs, non–prescribed drugs and personal health supplies bought in retail stores. Drugs prescribed in hospitals and in other institutions are *not* included in the 'drugs' category, but are included as part of expenditures in 'hospital' or 'other institutions' categories.

2 This tax-free benefit, or "tax-expenditure subsidy" is thus of greater value to people in higher tax brackets, *i.e.* with higher incomes.

3 The current trend from full-to part-time work, and from permanent to conditional or contracted employment, may then put in question the future extent of private coverage.

4 Bill C-91 was passed into law and is now known as the *Patent Act Amendment Act*, 1992.

5 Compulsory licensing refers to the system whereby a licence was granted by the Commissioner of Patents permitting the licensee to import, make, use or sell a patented invention pertaining to a medicine. Drug manufacturers granted a licence would pay royalties (determined by the Commissioner) to the holder of the patent. Bill C-91 abolished Canada's innovative compulsory licensing system, effectively extended the brand name companies' monopoly and ensured that a brand name product would be protected from generic competition until the patents on the products had expired.

6 Morgan, Steven G. 1997. "Issues for Canadian Pharmaceutical Policy".

7 The Patented Medicine Prices Review Board reports that under its review, prices of new drugs have increased at a slower pace than the consumer price index. But the normal pricing pattern over the "life cycle" of a prescription drug is that it enters the market at a high price, then remains stable or drifts downward as alternatives appear. The key questions are, at what price does the drug enter, and does its price in fact decline?

8 These would obviously include, but should not be restricted to, the Medical Research Council of Canada.

9 The PMPRB is an independent quasi-judicial body created by Parliament in 1987 under the *Patent Act*. It is mandated to regulate the prices charged by manufacturers of patented medicines to ensure that they are not excessive. The Board does not regulate the prices of non–patented drugs, including generic drugs sold under compulsory licences, and has no jurisdiction over prices charged by wholesalers or retailers or pharmacists' fees (PMPRB, 1996).

10 Personal communication with officials of the *Régie de l'Assurance-maladie du Quebec*.

11 As drugs are becoming a more important part of our health care system, allowance for increased expenditures has been made. Due to the high profitability of the pharmaceutical sector, as well as the research issues, and inefficient and inappropriate use described above, some degree of cost control is warranted.

12 Serious efforts by payers to manage pharmaceutical utilization and to control costs involve simultaneous intrusions on the profits of the drug industry and on the professional autonomy of physicians. As Margaret Thatcher would say, "There is no alternative." Not surprisingly, most payers have chosen to duck the issue by choosing cost-shifting policies and deferring the problem to someone else's watch.

13 The United States is an obvious exception. Over the last two decades, providers of all forms of health care have become increasingly active in all forms of competitive marketing. This has added materially to the overall costs of care, to pay both for the marketing activity itself, and for the resulting increases in utilization. There is no evidence of corresponding improvements in health status; nor should one expect any.

14 In this context, prescription drugs mean drugs classified as such under the *Food and Drugs Act* as well as other medically necessary drugs generally covered by public and private plans (e.g. insulin, nitroglycerin) for which a physician script may be required by the insurer.

15 See Kennedy (1997). Public policy has effectively made doctors responsible for the level of drugs prescribed. Any prescription levels above the regional medication budget cap are compensated by a diminution of doctors' revenue.

16 An indicator of the success of such "PBMs" may be that they are now being bought by drug manufacturers.

References

Baird, Patricia A. "Funding Medical and Health–Related Research in the Public Interest." *Canadian Medical Association Journal, 155, 3 (1996): 299–301.*

Canada. Health Canada. *National Health Expenditures in Canada, 1975–1994.* Full Report (January), and unpublished supplementary tabulations. Ottawa, 1996.

_____. National Forum on Health. *Report on Dialogue with Canadians.* Ottawa, July 1996.

_____. *Report on Dialogue: Seeking Solutions to Health and Health Care.* Ottawa, July 1996.

_____. "Creating a Culture of Evidence–Based Decision Making." *Canada Health Action: Building on the Legacy,* Vol. II. Ottawa, 1997.

_____. "Striking a Balance Working Group Synthesis Report." *Canada Health Action: Building on the Legacy,* Vol. II. Ottawa, 1997.

Coambes, R.B., P. Jensen, M. Hao Her, B. S. Ferguson, J. L. Jarry, J. S. Wong, and R. V. Abrahamsohn. *Review of the Literature on the Prevalence, Consequences, and Health Costs of Noncompliance and Inappropriate Use of Prescription Medication in Canada.* Prepared for the Pharmaceutical Manufacturers Association of Canada. University of Toronto Press, 1995.

CROP Conseil Inc. *Drug Benefit Programs in Canada.* Montreal, 1995.

Davidson, W., W. Molloy, G. Somers and M. Bédard. "Relation between physician characteristics and prescribing for elderly people in New Brunswick." *Canadian Medical Association Journal,* 150, 6 (1994): 917–20.

Kennedy, W. "Managing Pharmaceutical Expenditures: How Canada Compares." International Comparison Series Paper. *Papers Commissioned by the National Forum on Health.* Ottawa, 1997 (in press).

Lexchin, J. "Canadian Marketing Codes: How Well Are They Controlling Pharmaceutical Promotion?" *International Journal of Health Services,* 24,1 (1994).

_____. "Income Class and Pharmaceutical Expenditures in Canada: 1964–1990." *Canadian Journal of Public Health,* 87, 1 (1996): 46–50.

Morgan, S. "Issues for Canadian Pharmaceutical Policy." *Papers Commissioned by the National Forum on Health*. Ottawa, 1997 (in press).

Patented Medicine Prices Review Board. *Eighth Annual Report: For the Year Ended December 31, 1995*. Ottawa, 1996.

Québec. Assemblée nationale. *Loi sur l'assurance–médicaments et modifiant diverses dispositions législatives*. Éditeur officiel du Québec, 1996.

Report of the Committee of Experts on Drug Insurance. *Drug Insurance, Possible Approaches*. Bibliothèque nationale du Québec, 1996.

Tamblyn R. and R. Perreault. "Encouraging the Wise Use of Prescription Medication by Older Adults." *Papers Commissioned by the National Forum on Health*. Ottawa, 1997 (in press).

Wivell, M.K., and D. A. O'Fallon. "Drug Overpromotion: When Is a Warning Not a Warning?" *Trial*, 82, 11 (1992): 21-27.

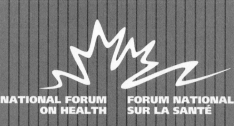

NATIONAL FORUM
ON HEALTH

FORUM NATIONAL
SUR LA SANTÉ

An Overview
of Women's
Health

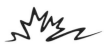

Preface

This paper draws on a variety of important works:

■ 30 papers on the determinants of health commissioned by the National Forum on Health

■ 27 papers prepared for the Canada–USA Forum on Women's Health held in August, 1996

■ A report on the dialogue with Canadians carried out by the National Forum on Health over the past two years

■ Material prepared by Health Canada to set a context for the work of the recently formed Centres of Excellence for Women's Health

The purpose of this paper is to provide information about key aspects and issues in women's health that have been identified in the scholarly papers referred to above and have been considered by the Forum's working groups.

Contents

Preface

The Context of Women's Health 3

What Makes Women Healthy or Unhealthy? 5

    Women, Income Distribution and Work. 5

    Violence in Women's Lives 6

    Women and Social Support 9

    Determinants of Reproductive Health. 9

    Personal Lifestyle Practices 11

    Gender as a Determinant of Health 11

Special Populations 12

    Aboriginal Women. 12

    Other Minority Women 13

    Lone–Parent Mothers 14

Women and Health Services 14

    Health Promotion 14

    Primary and Acute Care 15

    Effect of Health Care Reform on Women 16

    Women and Health Research 17

    Women in Leadership Roles 17

Implications for Policies and Programs 18

References 20

The Context of Women's Health

The 1995 Beijing Platform for Action states, "The major barrier for women to the achievement of the highest attainable standard of health is inequality, both between women and men and among women" (United Nations, 1995). Thus, countering the historical and systemic oppression of women must be foremost in our minds as we work to influence policy and practice at all levels: in government, in health services and in communities. This is confirmed in Canada in the Canadian Charter of Rights and Freedoms, sections 15 and 28.

While women in Canada enjoy far more equality than their sisters in many other countries, they continue to experience inequities in their lives. Inequality is manifested in the serious level of violence against women and the uneven workloads that occur in intimate and family relationships. In the workplace, it is manifested in unequal pay and benefits, a disproportionate share of low-level and part-time work and sexual harassment. In medicine and health, it is manifested in the under-attention given to female-specific diseases, in research with men that is generalized to women and in the over-medicalization of natural reproductive processes.

The Women's Health Interschool Curriculum Committee of Ontario has provided an important statement about women's health: "Women's health involves women's emotional, social, cultural, spiritual and physical well-being, and it is determined by the social, political and economic context of women's lives as well as by biology" (Phillips, 1995). This broad definition is in keeping with a population health approach that sees women as individuals and as a social group whose health is critically and intimately related to the conditions under which they live, learn, work and play. It also recognizes the diversity and validity of women's life experiences and women's own beliefs about health. Every woman should be provided with the opportunity to achieve, sustain and maintain health, as defined by that woman herself, to her full potential.

To understand women's health in context is to recognize that policies and programs in health and other sectors must squarely address the economic, social and political realities of women's lives. When economic inequity is defined as an issue with relevance to health, then progressive tax reform, a secure social safety net and health promotion activities become social policy goals.

While "sex" refers to the biological differences between men and women, "gender" takes into account the socially mediated differences as well. Gender includes the full range of attitudes, feelings, values, behaviours and activities that society ascribes to the two sexes on a differential basis.

In recent years, the Canadian Institute of Advanced Research, the Premier's Council (Ontario), Status of Women Canada and others have helped to advance our understanding of what makes people healthy or unhealthy by pulling together the research findings on the determinants of health. In addition, the National Forum on Health commissioned 30 papers on various aspects of the determinants of health. Unfortunately, there is little gender analysis in any of these sources.

It has been argued that gender should be added to the list of key determinants of health (along with education, income, social support, healthy child development, etc.). This addition would help planners, policy makers and programmers avoid inappropriate or inaccurate generalizations about "people" when gender differences are significant for health; it would ensure that these differences are taken into account. For example, the effects of low socioeconomic status or employment status may affect women's health differently than they do men's health.

Within the health care system, gendered norms have played out in the long-standing preoccupation of the system with women's reproductive and maternal functions. This has resulted in the medicalization of natural life occurrences such as the onset of menses, childbirth and menopause; a tendency to attribute women's mental health to hormones rather than living conditions; and, the development of programs that are more concerned with the health of an anticipated child than with the health of the woman herself. Ironically, over-medicalization of some aspects of women's health co-exists with the neglect of other key health issues specific to women (e.g., osteoporosis, pre-menstrual syndrome, nausea during pregnancy, breast cancer). In addition, the bulk of medical research has been done on men and generalized to women. This has led to insufficient attention being paid to the effects of some drugs and medical interventions on women.

The women's health movement has spearheaded a number of community-based approaches to health care that place a high priority on health promotion, disease prevention, information sharing and shared decision-making. These activities are chronically underfunded and in danger of disappearing with cutbacks in health care.

Finally, although women constitute the majority of workers in the formal and informal health care system, and many more women are now entering the medical profession than ever before, they hold fewer leadership positions than men. Generally, they are under represented among those who determine policy direction, manage large facilities and perform the gatekeeper functions in the system.

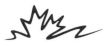

What Makes Women Healthy or Unhealthy?

Women, Income Distribution and Work

Income affects a woman's access to education, child care, some health care and types of employment, her actual or potential dependence on welfare payments, the safety of her neighbourhood, and her ability to obtain good affordable housing and nutrition for herself and her children.

Women are at greater risk of poverty than men, and women from Canada's Aboriginal communities are at particularly high risk: 33% (versus 17% of other Canadian women) have incomes below Statistics Canada's low income cutoff (Kaufert, 1996). Aboriginal women are less likely to be employed and to have completed high school. The burden of poverty and racism on their lives is reflected in the higher mortality rates of their children and their own shortened life expectancy. Racism and poverty are also key factors in the lives of the nine percent of Canadian women who belong to a visible minority group. They earn less than other Canadian women, and 28% have incomes below the cutoff point. Their rates of unemployment are higher and they are more likely to work in semi-skilled occupations (Kaufert, 1996).

Women's earnings are lower than men's at all levels of educational attainment. In 1994, women were less likely to be employed than men (52% versus 65%) and considerably

more likely to be working part-time (26% versus nine percent) (Statistics Canada, 1995). Part-time employment carries fewer benefits (e.g., pension rights), is more vulnerable to layoffs, is less likely to be unionized and is associated with higher levels of stress.

All but 14% of women work in service industries rather than in the production of goods. In 1994, 70% of women (versus 31% of men) were working in teaching, nursing and health-related occupations, clerical positions, or sales and service (Statistics Canada, 1995). Only seven percent of men report to a woman, but women are almost equally likely to report to either a man or a woman (Kaufert, 1996). Thus, women generally earn less than men, are less likely to be in a position of power than men and enjoy fewer career opportunities than men.

There are five factors that compromise women's health and well-being in the workplace:

■ *The relationship between lack of control and poor health* for both women and men has been well documented. The Framingham Study reported a relationship between coronary heart disease among women and a stressful clerical work environment (Hall, 1989). More recent research has linked musculoskeletal disorders and various forms of stress-related illness with the working conditions of women, particularly in the poultry processing and garment industries. High levels of depression have been associated with computer processing (Kaufert, 1996). Thus, women are disadvantaged relative to men in terms of job satisfaction because they are more likely to work in situations affording them little control over the pace and content of their tasks.

■ *Women work two shifts* — from 9:00 to 5:00 at work and 5:00 to 9:00 at home. Women's increased participation in the labour force overlaps with their extensive involvement in caregiving, adding considerable strain to their lives. By 1992, 61.4% of women were employed outside of the home, and 75% of mothers with children under 12 were working for pay. However, research reveals that the division of home labour in two-partner families has remained virtually unchanged over the years. Women continue to spend significantly more time than men on housework and the care of children and elderly relatives. A 1994 national survey of over 2,000 Canadian adults revealed that more than 25% of employed women thought that they did not have a good balance between their jobs and time spent with their families. About 20% of these women believed that family responsibilities and difficulties experienced trying to balance job and family demands had limited their career advancement (Frederick, 1995).

■ *Environmental occupational risks* may be especially harmful to women's health. Attention to women's reproductive health should not be limited to fetal protection but should also include attention to fertility, sexuality, early menopause and menstrual disorders. It is important that pregnant and nursing women be given rapid access to up-to-date information on occupational and environmental risks that may affect them, as well as to programs for the protection of their health. Methods should also

be developed for diminishing exposure to chemicals in jobs usually done by women, e.g., hairdressers, cleaners and laboratory technicians (Messing, 1996).

■ *Sexual harassment* is now accepted as a mental health issue affecting women in the course of their work. An estimated 42% to 80% of women are sexually harassed at some time in their working lives. Women who have been harassed exhibit a variety of stress-related illnesses including weight loss, diarrhea, sleeplessness, headaches, fatigue, loss of feelings of self-worth, acute depression, anxiety and nervousness.

■ *Job insecurity* is higher for women than for men because more work part-time or take time off with young children (thus losing their seniority in the workplace). Research on the impact of unemployment suggests that men and women experience the same degree of anxiety and loss of self-esteem and are as likely to be depressed.

The work-related determinants of health that particularly affect women can be addressed by reducing job pace, implementing more flexible and supportive family-friendly terms of employment (work hours, pay level, overtime, benefits), providing subsidized child care, enhancing job security, improving safety standards, putting an end to sexual harassment, increasing employee control in female-dominated jobs, encouraging men to do more child care and housework and improving social support.

Violence in Women's Lives

Gender-based violence includes intimate partner violence, sexual assault, sexual harassment, sexual and other forms of child abuse, marital rape, date rape, elder abuse and female genital mutilation. The most common of these is violence perpetrated by one's partner.

One half of Canadian women over 16 years of age, report violence at the hands of an intimate partner at some point during their lives (Statistics Canada, 1993). Women are over four times more likely to be injured by their male partner than in a motor vehicle accident. Stalking and harassment after separation are commonplace. Women are more likely to be killed by their partner or ex-partner than by anyone else in the community (Sudermann and Jaffe, 1997).

Women who have been assaulted often suffer from severe psychological and physical health conditions. The impact of sexual abuse and gender-based violence on women at any age may include unwanted pregnancy, miscar-riage, sexually transmitted disease, HIV infection, pregnancy complications and other gynaecological problems. The psychological effects include trauma, fear, anxiety, depression and suicide attempts (Kinnon and Hanvey, 1996). Forty-three percent of injuries afflicted by spouses require medical attention (Statistics Canada, 1993). Dating violence and the sexual assault of young women have been linked to poor self-esteem and eating disorders (Gallers and Lawrence, 1990).

Aside from the immediate risks to physical and psychological well-being, violence against women is estimated to cost the Canadian econ-omy at least $4 billion per year in the justice, health, social service and employment sectors. This includes over $408 million in direct health care costs (Greaves et al, 1995).

The most extensive study on child sexual abuse in Canada found that 53% of females and 31% of males had been victims of unwanted sexual acts and that 80% of these incidents occurred when they were children or adolescents (Committee on Sexual Offences Against Children and Youth, 1984). Most professionals, however, believe that this is an underestimate. Violence during childhood can deeply interfere with learning, and sexual abuse is cited as a common reason why girls leave home and drop out of school (Kinnon and Hanvey, 1996).

Children who witness violence are at high risk for emotional and behavioural adjustment problems. Boys in particular are at risk to repeat violent behaviours they learn through observing their fathers (National Clearinghouse on Family Violence, 1992).

Violence in relationships often begins during early courtship and dating relationships; young women are overwhelmingly the victims of these forms of violence. In a 1993 national survey of university students, 20% of men reported that they had been sexually abusive, 18% of men were physically abusive, and 80% of men reported being psychologically abusive within the same time period (DeKeseredy and Kelley, 1993).

Four determining factors related to gender are particularly important in providing effective efforts to address violence against women (Kinnon and Hanvey, 1996):

■ *The social context of power imbalances:* People who lack power in society are the most likely victims of violence because they lack the means to resist abuse and to escape from dangerous situations.

- *Attitudes and values:* Violence is condoned by Canadian social values that see violence as a natural expression of aggression or an inevitable result of stress, anger and frustration. One in five people think that wife abuse is acceptable, and most people do not want to get involved (Strauss, 1989). Gender stereotyping of females and males in television, radio, video games and other entertainment media reinforces and condones both subtle and overt violence against women.

- *Isolation and alienation:* Child poverty, school failure and other blocked opportunities for youth are major risk factors for young men to become persistent offenders. The loss of a sense of community because of greater mobility, larger urban centres and the changing nature of family is also creating a sense of isolation. These factors may result in a greater concern for individual survival and a lesser sense of social responsibility for others (Canadian Public Health Association, 1994) .

- *Vulnerable individuals and groups:* Particular groups of girls and women are more vulnerable to violence than others:

  - Girls and young women are especially vulnerable to abuse by parents, adult caregivers, acquaintances and boyfriends.

  - About 80% of women with a disability will be sexually assaulted in their lifetime (Stimpson and Best, 1991).

- Women with a household income under $15,000 are twice as likely to be battered as women in general (Canadian Centre for Justice Statistics, 1994).

- One in 10 older people experience abuse and at least two-thirds of these are women (Canadian Panel on Violence Against Women, 1993).

- In many Aboriginal communities, economic changes, cultural losses and male domination of political life have compromised the traditional social structure. Historical abuse in church, schools and high levels of alcohol abuse exacerbate the problem. Among Aboriginal women, the rates of abuse may be as high as 80%, and in some communities all women have a history of abuse (Ontario Native Women's Association, 1989).

- Immigrant women, women of colour, refugee women, live-in domestic workers and women from linguistic minorities often encounter barriers in gaining access to appropriate services and therefore bear a greater burden from violence than other women (Shin, 1992).

In general, government policies have not dealt effectively with socioeconomic issues related to violence such as economic independence for women, adequate income levels for families and for women and children who leave violent relationships, safer indoor and outdoor environments, and so on. Current reductions in spending on social, educational and health programs at all levels threaten progress made in addressing the socioeconomic determinants of violence.

Strategies for putting an end to violence against women and girls must include concrete actions to enhance the status of women in Canada and to address sources of inequality and discrimination. This approach will require coordinated efforts among all sectors of society and all governments at the national, provincial, territorial and local levels. Community-wide involvement is also important. Women want an approach to prevention that recognizes women's strengths, is community-based, is empowering and multifaceted, works with women's children and partners, and gives women the tools and support they need to build lives free of violence.

Developing a network between police and community resources that provides services for women and abused children is critical. How services conceptualize the significance of the trauma of witnessing violence is also important. Recent innovations, including school-based violence prevention programs and specialized group counselling programs, offer some hope for longer-term reduction in violence.

There is abundant evidence that violence is often overlooked in primary health care contacts. A recent study of Ontario doctors indicated that, by their own estimate, they identified fewer than 50% of abused patients in their own practices (Canadian Public Health Association, 1994). Primary health care has an essential role to play in identifying risk factors for violence, providing early intervention and treatment, and providing crisis and on-going support to victims, abusers and others who are affected.

Women and Social Support

Family support is critical to married women's success in the workplace. Currently, employed women experience greater demands and stressors than their male counterparts due to the double burden of work and family responsibilities (Kaufert, 1996).

While social support and interaction are important at all ages, they are especially important for healthy aging. Older women are more likely than older men to be interested in and comfortable with social interaction, but many older women are constrained by caregiving responsibilities with a spouse or relative who is ill.

In recent years, women have formed support groups to share information and resources about specific health problems and to offer each other emotional support. In some cases, these groups have also become important catalysts for research and advocacy. Research now shows that being involved in a breast cancer support group not only improves quality of life but significantly increases length of survival.

Determinants of Reproductive Health

A number of past and present legal controls on women involve their sexual and reproductive processes. These controls provide evidence of underlying and deeply entrenched beliefs about women and childbearing in general. At present there are no statutory prohibitions against abortion in Canada, but funding and access are uneven across the country (e.g., there are no abortion services on Prince

Edward Island). Abortion services remain an uncomfortable, value-laden issue for governments. Those who provide abortion services are often threatened and besieged.

One of the most contentious issues over the past several years has been the management and regulation of new reproductive technologies. In 1993, the Canadian government released the report of the Royal Commission on New Reproductive Technologies. The report adopted an "ethic of care", which consists of eight guiding principles: individual autonomy, equality, respect for human life and dignity, protection of the vulnerable, non-commercialization of reproduction, appropriate use of resources, accountability, and balancing of individual and collective interests (Royal Commission on New Reproductive Technologies, 1993).

In response, in June of 1996, the federal government tabled legislation in the House of Commons that would prohibit certain practices such as germ line genetic alteration, cloning, sale of gametes and embryos, and "surrogacy" arrangements. In addition, the federal government also tabled a discussion paper outlining a legislative regime that would deal with other reproductive and genetic practices that should be allowed, but regulated.

Other reproductive health issues that are affected by broad sociopolitical factors include the following:

■ Sexually transmitted diseases and infections affect women differently from men. Men have earlier detection rates and experience less long-term damage, particularly in relation to infertility. Being poor, living on the street and working in the sex trade increases a woman's likelihood of infection (McDonald, 1996).

■ Women have not comprised a large percentage of HIV and AIDS cases in Canada to date. However, there is growing concern that later diagnoses in women preclude early treatment. A related issue is the discrimination experienced by HIV- infected women in both research and treatment, together with ongoing discrimination within society at large. This discrimination will particularly affect immigrant women from countries where HIV infection is widespread. There are also concerns about adolescent women's and Aboriginal women's ability to negotiate condom use in male-dominated environments (McDonald, 1996).

■ A medical model of care emphasizing technological intervention has resulted in many women's deep dissatisfaction with their birthing experience. In response, some physicians and hospitals have taken steps to naturalize and improve birthing practices. An alternative is the midwifery model, which emphasizes holistic care and the woman's role as primary decision-maker. In response to consumer demands and demonstrated cost-effectiveness, a piecemeal process of official acceptance and regulation of midwifery is occurring on a province-by-province basis. It remains to be seen whether jurisdictions will implement a true midwifery model, as opposed to merely substituting lower-paid midwives for physicians within the existing medical model. The health care system must recognize birth care decisions as essential aspects of women's autonomy and affirm the understanding that health in pregnancy and birth includes emotional, social and cultural elements.

- The experience of menopause in women was, until recently, seriously misunderstood or dismissed. There is now a recognition of the need for more research on risk factors and more accessible screening procedures for specific groups of women with family histories of osteoporosis and heart disease. Hormone replacement therapy appears to offer many advantages. However, given the historical experience of women with various birth control pharmaceutical products, many women are sceptical about these drugs.

- In the Great Lakes Basin and other environmentally damaged areas of the country, women are profoundly concerned about their reproductive health and the health of future generations. These concerns include the effects of contaminants on the fetus and on breast-feeding and the effects of environmental toxins, pollutants and nuclear fallout on cancer rates, endometriosis and other reproductive problems (Bertell, 1996).

- Women with low socioeconomic status are at higher risk for preterm births and for delivering low birth weight babies. However, a variety of programs have demonstrated that the social and health contexts for childbearing in severely socially disadvantaged families can be improved. These programs include home-visiting programs designed to enhance prenatal care and parenting practices, and the provision of nutritional counselling, social support and food supplements for high-risk pregnant women (Steinhauer, 1997).

Personal Lifestyle Practices

National data for youth aged 15 to 19 indicate that, for the first time, more girls (25%) than boys (19%) are smoking (Statistics Canada, 1994-95). The reasons for this increase are largely societal: pressure on young women to cope with high levels of stress and to be thin and sexy. Adolescent women are also engaging in intercourse at an earlier age and with a greater number of partners. Seen in the context of unequal gender relations and low self-esteem, it is not surprising that young women engage in risky behaviour even when they understand the possible consequences of such activity. Sex education programs must address gender role socialization and power imbalances between men and women if they are to be successful (McDonald, 1996).

Stress and lack of time are persistent themes in studies that have asked women about why they smoke, misuse alcohol or medication, or do not exercise. Efforts to change lifestyle behaviours need to recognize that the socio-economic conditions of women's lives greatly affect their behaviours. Smoking may be a symptom of other stresses; poor eating habits may reflect a lack of capacity to purchase healthy foods (Cohen and Sinding, 1996).

Gender as a Determinant of Health

In view of what we know about the determinants of health, questions arise about how these determinants of health influence the lives of Canadian women differently than men. Although it may appear that women are healthier than men, because they live longer than men, other socioeconomic indicators suggest that this may not be the case. On the one hand, in comparison to men, women in Canada earn significantly less, suffer more chronic and disabling diseases, are more likely to head a lone-parent family and present lower rates of self-esteem but, nevertheless live longer than men. On the other hand, men have higher prevalence of risk-taking behaviour such as accidents, substance abuse, criminal activities, and suicide.

How do we account for the large gap in the average life expectancy age between the sexes?

This paradox is not well understood. Biological factors associated with being female may explain only part of the paradox. It has been hypothesised that the importance women give to networking and personal relationships or the multiple social roles in women's lives may have a buffering effect to protect them from the negative stress in their lives. But, these and other hypotheses remain speculation at the present time. Our limited understanding of these significant factors in women's lives demands more research, both quantitative and qualitative, on the non-medical determinants of women's health.

Special Populations

Women who are members of particular cultural groups such as Aboriginal women, lone parent mothers, women with disabilities, lesbians, women of colour, and other special populations, face particular health issues. A few examples are discussed below.

Aboriginal Women

Aboriginal women face a heightened risk of health problems in a wide range of areas (Dion Stout, 1996).

- In 1986, the life expectancy at birth for Aboriginal women was 71 years, compared to 81 for non-Aboriginal women.

- The suicide rate for Aboriginal adolescent girls is eight times the national average.

- The diabetes rate among Aboriginal peoples is 10 times the Canadian rate and is generally higher for females.

- Rates of cardiovascular and respiratory diseases, eye and ear infections and dental and gastrointestinal problems are all much higher among Aboriginal women than in the female population in general. Aboriginal women suffer higher rates of cervical cancer, sexually transmitted disease and cirrhosis of the liver than their non-Aboriginal counterparts.

- Many Aboriginal women and children are forced to relocate to the city on account of the violence they are experiencing in their homes. Their marginalized socioeconomic status pushes them into substandard, unsafe or crowded housing.

- Poor socioeconomic conditions worsen the life chances and health status of Canadian Aboriginal women. Poverty undermines one's sense of self-worth and is correlated with poor nutrition, smoking and other unhealthy practices.

- Aboriginal women often find mainstream health systems alien, confusing and insensitive to Aboriginal cultural values.

Aboriginal people have sought to come to terms with the many traumas that they have endured. This has led to an emphasis on the role of healing as the means by which individual and collective development can be undertaken in harmony with the environment. With the transfer of control over health care services to First Nations communities, and the growing acceptance of the value of traditional forms of medicine, there is reason for (cautious) optimism about the future direction that Aboriginal women's health will take in this country. However, for Aboriginal women to achieve their full health potential, there must be a sustained commitment on the part of all concerned parties to tackle both the effects of ill health and its underlying causes.

Other Minority Women

The main health issues for immigrant and racial minority women in Canada include the following (Simms, 1996):

- isolation from mainstream society created by differing cultural values

- cultural belief systems and practices that create serious barriers for women in understanding, gaining access to and interacting with the health care system

- lack of access to culturally sensitive health care services

- problems of professional accreditation that prevent highly qualified women from participating in the health care professions

- the inability of large numbers of immigrant and refugee women to speak English or French, which is seen as the major obstacle to gaining access to social services

- the underrepresentation of immigrant and racial minority women in the health care professions and on the boards of directors of hospitals, universities and other major institutions that train personnel and set policies that determine the level and type of health care

- compromised mental health due to the stigmatization of their immigration, their socioeconomic status, racism and marginalization.

The challenge for health practitioners is to emphasize the strengths of the minority populations they serve. What is needed is a health care system that has ways of incorporating learning, knowledge and expertise from these communities to meet the educational, therapeutic, preventive and healing challenges that are inherent within the dimensions of a multicultural Canada.

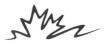

Lone-Parent Mothers

In Canada, approximately 60% of all single parents, the great majority of whom are women, live below the poverty line. For parents aged 16 to 24, the percentage jumps to 80 (National Council of Welfare, 1992). While lone-parent families comprise 13% of all Canadian families, they comprise 19% of Inuit families, 24% of on-reserve Indian families and 30% of off-reserve Indian families. Although the reasons for the high incidence of lone parenthood among Aboriginal peoples are complex, the effects on the health of mothers and children almost inevitably include the various illnesses associated with marginalized socioeconomic status (Dion Stout, 1996).

The national rate for adolescent pregnancy was 41 per 1,000 in 1991 (Statistics Canada, 1995). Early or unintended pregnancy among young women has serious health and socioeconomic implications for these women, their children and society as a whole. Eighty per cent to 90 percent of pregnant adolescents who bear children to term choose to raise them. Of these, 50% to 70% will quit school, and about 60% will go on welfare (National Council of Welfare, 1992). Interrupted education and lack of adequate child care and other social support systems translate into lower employment rates and poverty. Social stigma also hurts health. Some studies state that the lack of a husband is less important than how society decides to treat women with children but without a partner. Current changes in the ideological and political framework of North America have created a very negative image of the single mother and threaten her access to social support (Kaufert, 1996).

Women and Health Services

A gendered approach to health services extending from health promotion to acute and continuing care is necessary, because women make up the majority of health care workers and consumers and serve as the "health guardians" of their families.

Health Promotion

Health promotion is "the process of enabling people to increase control over and to improve their health" (World Health Organization, 1986). It particularly aims at effective and concrete public participation which is a cornerstone of the women's health movement.

In spite of the rhetoric of health reform, health promotion and disease prevention strategies have remained secondary to health care delivery. Indeed, in some cases, objectives in other policy areas have been shown to be in direct opposition to health promotion objectives. For example, public efforts to curb the influence of the tobacco industry suffered setbacks through a court decision permitting the reinstatement of wide-scale advertising and the political decision to reduce taxes on tobacco to address smuggling. This has led to a dramatic increase in smoking among young women. Rates of lung cancer among women (which has already surpassed breast cancer as the main cancer killer of women) will inevitably rise as a result.

If women's health and well-being are to be enhanced, intersectoral population health promotion efforts that address the basic determinants of health must be supported (Thurston and O'Connor, 1996).

Primary and Acute Care

Women have identified the following key issues in health care delivery:

■ differentials of power and authority between the roles of both male and female doctors and patients

■ sexist and paternalistic attitudes that may influence interactions between male doctors and female patients or result in abuse

■ severe time constraints on most medical encounters which serve to limit communication between patient and caregiver

■ lack of sufficient information to make informed decisions about proposed treatments

■ fragmented care, which prompts a patient to feel that she is no more than the sum of her body parts

■ inappropriate uses of technologies, drugs and devices

■ added barriers for lesbians, women with disabilities, women from diverse cultures, rural and farm women and survivors of abuse

■ the "two patient" theory of service delivery to pregnant women, which creates a false opposition between a pregnant woman and her foetus.

Women have pressured mainstream health institutions to change by advocating for birthing rooms, interpreters in hospitals, midwifery, non-sexist curricula in medical schools and more home care services. They have also organized and supported a broad range of creative models of community-based health services. These include:

■ community health centres offering primary care, health promotion and a variety of social services, from counselling to help with housing

■ battered women's shelters

■ community kitchens

■ women's centres providing health information, parenting support and nutrition programs

■ reproductive health projects serving the needs of women in immigrant and refugee communities

■ health promotion resources and programs providing health information, services and supports geared to women's needs.

As criteria for appropriate care are developed, women's concerns about inappropriate and insensitive approaches to care (such as unnecessary hysterectomies or ignoring early symptoms of heart disease in women) must be considered. Determining the appropriate provider for particular health services is also necessary for good, cost-effective care. Some services and examinations provided by family physicians or even specialists can be performed by other health providers such as nurses, nurse practitioners, and nutritionists, who may also take the time to pass on more specific health information to clients.

Determining the right settings in which to deliver particular services is also key to designing appropriate care. Isolated communities may have creative solutions to the need for health and wellness services. For example, the Innulitsivik Maternity Facility trained local Inuit midwives to perform deliveries and do health promotion among the community, particularly with high-risk teens. The majority of women are no longer flown south for birthing, thus avoiding the pain of dislocation from family and community members.

Effect of Health Care Reform on Women

In most provinces, reform strategies have concentrated on reducing hospital costs through closing, amalgamating and centralizing facilities, and cutting staff and services, most notably nurses and nurses aides. Chronic patients are being moved from hospitals to community care. Limits have been put on the length of stay per patient, and new standards for procedures result in much earlier discharges. Some of these policies, such as the early discharge of new mothers and the simultaneous withdrawal of health support, have serious effects on the health of both mother and child.

Other aspects of reform will have profound effects on women if community back-up services are not in place. When community and home care services are limited, women are expected to meet the need. Working women may be forced to take unpaid leave from their jobs or change to part- time work to care for family members who are chronically ill or recovering from an illness. Older women may become home bound and burdened with additional caregiving responsibilities. The physical and emotional effects of caregiving can be devastating. Ironically, they may also result in increased use of the health system by women. These costs must be included when measuring the real costs of health reform.

Women represent 80% of all Canadian health care workers and are experiencing a disproportionate amount of the layoffs and cutbacks to the health sector (Trudiver and Hall, 1996). There has also been a shift from full time to part time positions with no or limited job security and benefits.

Remaining staff must cope with increased workloads and tensions among co-workers. The impacts of restructuring on rural health care workers can be especially serious.

Health reform strategies in most provinces have also involved a move to pool regional resources under the auspices of regional health boards. In theory, regional boards are more responsive to residents' health needs and will reduce duplication of services through enhanced integration and an improved allocation of resources. However, if women are not equally represented on regional boards, this lack of diversity will hamper the capacity of regional health boards to address women's health issues and services.

Health reform should be a carefully planned process, based on analyzing successful health delivery models and assessing the strengths and weaknesses of past policies and structures. Provincial and federal governments must recognize that future cost-savings require significant expenditures now to address poverty and other major determinants of health. Reforms should include training in new roles and should use people's skills to redesign and address the many health and social service needs identified within a region. Home care, child day care, and respite and shorter term crisis services can be expanded, as can a host of public health and health promotion activities.

Women and Health Research

While women's health research in general receives insufficient funding, an additional problem is the disproportionately high amount of funding that is allocated to women's reproductive capacities. Pregnancy, reproduction, cancer and infections accounted for over 70% of research activities, while 16% of research was directed to the social and mental components of health. Further, there is little evidence of a balance between quantitative and qualitative methodologies, which allow women's own perspectives to be heard directly (Lefebvre, 1996).

The research community is increasingly recognizing the importance of directing funding to diseases unique to, more prevalent in or more serious in women. As more research is done on women's diseases, the historical assumption that clinical research findings can be generalized from men to women is becoming less and less acceptable in scientific terms. As well, the need to make research results apply to both sexes does not mean simply adding women as research subjects, but it involves gender sensitive research methodologies.

The enhancement of research that benefits Canadian women must include efforts to:

- define a research agenda that is gender sensitive and inclusive

- conduct interdisciplinary research involving both qualitative and quantitative methods

- ensure meaningful participation by women at every stage of the research process

- promote women researchers

- develop efficient and effective ways to transform the results of research into health policy (Lefebvre, 1996).

There are also new opportunities for policy-focused research on women's health through the five Centres of Excellence for Women's Health, recently funded by Health Canada. The Centres will not be involved in biomedical research but will encourage collaboration and participatory research among community-based women's health groups, service providers and academic researchers on many aspects of the social determinants of health, health reform policies and gender-specific models of care.

Women in Leadership Roles

If health leadership refers to the power to make and implement policy and control in training, practice and administration, then women as a group have been and continue to be underrepresented. Although the majority of health care workers are women, they are clustered in the lower paying, less powerful occupations and professions. In medicine, which has traditionally directed policy and

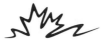

dominated institutions, the number of practitioners is slowly increasing, although the number of women in medical school has greatly increased and the demographics of the profession will be quite different in 20 years.

Implications for Policies and Programs

Women, like men, are a diverse group of people. Efforts to improve women's health must celebrate and pay attention to this diversity and give special recognition to the health needs of those women who are most in need. Initiatives must also address the various life stages and transitions that girls and women go through.

At the same time, from a health point of view, women in Canada—for a mix of social, political, cultural and biological reasons—probably share more in common with each other than they do with men.

This synthesis suggests that a broad population health strategy designed to improve the health and well-being of women in Canada needs to focus on the following:

1. Reducing power inequities that lead to social inequities and violence. Violence against women and poverty caused by inequalities in the workforce and the home are without doubt, the greatest causes of poor health among women.

2. Relieving women's double workload. Taxation and workplace policies that support caregiving and access to high-quality, low-cost child care are essential for the improved health of women and their families.

3. Ensuring the genuine participation of diverse communities of women in all areas of health research, planning and

service delivery, especially in areas related to reproductive health. Women's lack of influence in decision-making has a negative impact on health. Genuine recognition, including remuneration, must accompany women's contributions to health policy, planning, research and service delivery.

4. Supporting the efforts of Aboriginal women and women from minority communities to educate themselves, to create networks and to gain control over their health.

5. Supporting the development of women- and family-centred health services. This support includes increased emphasis on community health promotion and disease prevention initiatives as well as increased access to client-centred primary care. Currently, services of value to women are being curtailed; government spending cuts and structural adjustment activities may extend and deepen already existing gender inequities.

6. Guarding against the over-medicalization of women's health. Health services need to view women's reproductive functions as natural and healthy parts of life. It is also important to avoid the medicalization of issues that are related to the broader determinants of health. As we increasingly talk about violence as a health issue, we run the risk of focusing primarily on the medical impacts of violence, perhaps to the exclusion of other impacts. As well, if we think about violence as primarily a health issue, we think of health professionals as the group charged with defining what is important about violence, what constitutes violence, how violence should be addressed, and so on. In these ways,

the broad and complex roots and repercussions of sociopolitical issues risk being obscured (Cohen and Sinding, 1996). Initiatives to stop violence against girls and women must use an integrated approach that involves all of the key sectors at all levels.

7. Attending to the burden that health system reform represents for women. Health system reform—including the advent of new caregivers such as nurse practitioners and midwives, support for more citizen responsibility for personal health and health system decision-making, and an increased emphasis on health promotion—has the potential to benefit women. At the same time, early hospital discharge and the shifting of chronically ill people to the community without back-up services in place will mean that women will be required to take on disproportionate caregiving responsibilities they cannot afford and for which they may be ill equipped. "Community-based care" cannot become a euphemism for the conscription of women to provide unpaid health care services.

8. Providing increased support for gender and sex specific research, female health researchers (especially in applied research) and gender analyses of research results (in both medicine and the broad determinants of health).

9. Supporting women in leadership roles, that is decision-making and gatekeeping roles in health and health policy.

References

Bertell, R. *Environmental Impacts on the Health of Women in the Great Lakes Basin.* Paper prepared for the Canada-USA Forum on Women's Health. Ottawa: Health Canada, 1996.

Canada. Statistics Canada. National Population Health Survey. Original analysis, reported in *Report on the Health of Canadians.* Ottawa: Federal, Provincial and Territorial Advisory Committee on Population Health, 1994-95.

_____ .*Women in Canada: A Statistical Report*, 3rd edition. Ottawa, 1995.

_____ .*The Violence Against Women Survey.* Ottawa, 1993.

Capen, K. *Legal, Ethical and Legislative Issues and Women's Health in Canada.* Paper prepared for the Canada-USA Forum on Women's Health. Ottawa: Health Canada, 1996.

Canadian Centre for Justice Statistics. "Wife Assault: The Findings of a National Survey." *Juristat*, 14, 9 (1994).

Canadian Panel on Violence Against Women. *Changing the Landscape: Ending Violence, Achieving Equality.* Ottawa, 1993.

Canadian Public Health Association. *Violence in Society: A Public Health Perspective.* Ottawa, 1994.

Cohen, M. and C. Sinding. *Changing Concepts of Women's Health: Advocating for Change.* Paper prepared for Canada-USA Forum on Women's Health. Ottawa: Health Canada, 1996.

Committee on Sexual Offenses Against Children and Youth. *Sexual Offenses Against Children.* Ottawa, 1984.

DeKeseredy, W. and K. Kelley. "The Incidence and Prevalence of Woman Abuse in Canadian University and College Dating Relationships." *The Canadian Journal of Sociology.* 18, 2 (1993).

Dion Stout, M. *Aboriginal Canada: Women and Health.* Paper prepared for the Canada- USA Forum on Women's Health. Ottawa: Health Canada, 1996.

Frederick, J. "As Time Goes By ... Time Use of Canadians." *General Social Survey.* Ottawa: Statistics Canada, Catalogue No. 89-544E, 1995.

Gallers, J. and K. Lawrence. "Overcoming Post-Traumatic Stress Disorder in Adolescent Date Rape Survivors", in *Dating Violence: Young Women in Danger*, B. Levy (ed.). Seattle: Seal Press, 1990.

Greaves, L., O. Hankivsky, and J. Kingston-Riechers. *Selected Estimates of the Costs of Violence Against Women*. London, ON: London Centre for Research on Violence Against Women and Children, 1995.

Hall, E. "Gender, Work Control and Stress: A Theoretical Discussion and an Empirical Test." *International Journal of Health Services* 19 (1989).

Kaufert, P. *Gender as a Determinant of Health*. Paper prepared for the Canada-USA Forum on Women's Health. Ottawa: Health Canada, 1996.

Kinnon, D. and L. Hanvey. *Health Aspects of Violence Against Women: A Canadian Perspective*. Paper prepared for the Canada-USA Forum on Women's Health. Ottawa: Health Canada, 1996.

Lefebvre, Y. *Women's Health Research in Canada*. Paper prepared for the Canada-USA Forum on Women's Health. Ottawa: Health Canada, 1996.

McDonald, K. *Sexual and Reproductive Health and Rights in Canada*. Paper prepared for the Canada-USA Forum on Women's Health. Ottawa: Health Canada, 1996.

Messing, K. *Women and Occupational Health in Canada: A Critical Review and Discussion of Current Issues*. Paper prepared for the Canada-USA Forum on Women's Health. Ottawa: Health Canada, 1996.

National Clearinghouse on Family Violence. *Information Fact Sheet: Wife Abuse — The Impact on Children*. Ottawa: Health and Welfare Canada, 1992.

National Council of Welfare. *Poverty Profile: Update from 1991*. 12, 4 (1992): 6-10.

Ontario Native Women's Association. *Breaking Free: A Proposal for Change to Aboriginal Family Violence*. Thunder Bay, 1989.

Phillips, S. "The Social Context of Women's Health: Goals and Objectives for Medical Education." *Canadian Medical Association Journal*, 152, 4, (February 1995): 507.

Royal Commission on New Reproductive Technologies. *Proceed With Care: Final Report of the Royal Commission on New Reproductive Technologies*. Ottawa, 1993.

Shin, M. *Violence Against Immigrant and Visible Minority Women: Speaking with our Voice, Organizing from Our Experience*. Ottawa: National Organization of Immigrant and Visible Minority Women of Canada, 1992.

Simms, G. *Aspects of Women's Health from a Minority/Diversity Perspective*. Paper prepared for the Canada-USA Forum on Women's Health. Ottawa: Health Canada, 1996.

Steinhauer, Paul D. "Developing Resiliency in Children from Disadvantaged Populations." *Papers Commissioned by the National Forum on Health*. Ottawa, 1997 (in press).

Stimpson, L. and M.C. Best. *Courage Above All: Sexual Assault Against Women with Disabilities*. Toronto: Disabled Women's Network, 1991.

Strauss, M.A. Cited in *Family Violence Review: Prevention and Treatment of Abusive Behaviour* by B. Appleford. Ottawa: Correctional Services Canada, 1989.

Sudermann, M. and P. Jaffe. "Preventing Violence: School and Community-Based Strategies." *Papers Commissioned by the National Forum on Health*. Ottawa, 1997 (in press).

Thurston, W. and M. O'Connor. *Health Promotion for Women*. Paper prepared for the Canada-USA Forum on Women's Health. Ottawa: Health Canada, 1996.

Trudiver, S. and M. Hall. *Women and Health Service Delivery in Canada*. Paper prepared for the Canada-USA Forum on Women's Health. Ottawa: Health Canada, 1996.

United Nations. *Report of the 4th World Conference on Women (United Nations Platform for Action on Women's Equality)*. Beijing, 4-15 September. New York, 1995.

World Health Organization. *Ottawa Charter for Health Promotion*. Ottawa, 1986.

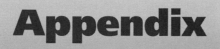

Appendix

National Forum on Health Publications

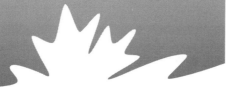

Forum Publications

Advancing the Dialogue on Health and Health Care: A Consultation Document. October 1996.

Health and Health Care Issues Summaries of Papers Commissioned by the National Forum on Health. February 1997.

InfoForum. Quarterly Newsletter. ISSN 1201-6853.

Let's Talk... About our Health and Health Care. November 1995.

Maintaining a National Health Care System: a Question of Principle(s)... and Money. February 1996.

National Forum on Health. Brochure. 1995.

The Public and Private Financing of Canada's Health System. September 1995.

Report on Dialogue: Seeking Solutions to Health and Health Care. July 1996.

Report on Dialogue with Canadians. July 1996.

Reporting... A one-year report on the National Forum on Health. December 1995.

Summary Report: Evidence-Based Decision Making: A Dialogue on Health Information. May 1995.

Summary Report: Changing the Health Care System - A Consumer Perspective. June 1995.

What Determines Health? Summaries of a Series of Papers on the Determinants of Health Commissioned by the National Forum on Health. Second Edition, September 1996.

Video:

The Future of Our Health and Health System: Stories of Choice. September 1996.

Papers Commissioned by the National Forum on Health

(Note: These papers will be published in 1997.)

Values Working Group

Ekos Research Associates Inc. and Earnscliffe Research and Communications. "Research on Canadian Values in Relation to Health and the Health Care System."

Leroux, Thérese, Sonia Le Bris and Bartha Maria Knoppers. "The Feasibility of a National Canadian Ethics Advisory Committee: Points to Consider."

Determinants of Health Working Group

Anisef, Paul. "Making the Transition from School to Employment."

Avison, William R. "The Health Consequences of Unemployment."

Bagley, Christopher and Wilfreda E. Thurston. "Decreasing Child Sexual Abuse."

Bennett, Kathryn and David R. Offord. "Schools, Mental Health and Life Quality."

Bertrand, Jane E. "Enriching the Preschool Experiences of Children."

Breen, Mary J. "Promoting Literacy, Improving Health."

Caputo, Tullio and Katherine Kelly. "Improving the Health of Street/Homeless Youth."

Chappell, Neena L. "Maintaining and Enhancing Independence and Well-being in Old Age."

Dyck, Ronald J., Brian L. Mishara and Jennifer White. "Suicide in Children, Adolescents and Seniors: Key Findings and Policy Implications."

Fralick, Pamela C. "Youth, Substance Abuse and the Determinants of Health."

Godin, Gaston and Francine Michaud. "STD and AIDS Prevention Among Young People."

Gottlieb, Benjamin H. "Protecting and Promoting the Well-being of Family Caregivers."

Gottlieb, Benjamin H. "Strategies to Promote the Optimal Development of Canada's Youth."

Hamel, Pierre. "Community Solidarity and Local Development: A New Perspective for Building Socio-political Compromise."

Lord, John and Peggy Hutchison. "Living with a Disability in Canada: Toward Autonomy and Integration."

McDaniel, Susan A. "Toward Healthy Families."

Marshall, Victor W. and Philippa J. Clarke. "Facilitating the Transition from Employment to Retirement."

Morrongiello, Barbara. A. "Preventing Unintentional Injuries Among Children."

Nahmiash, Daphne. "Preventing, Reducing and Stopping the Abuse and Neglect of Older Adults in Canadian Communities."

O'Brien Cousins, Sandra. "Promoting Active Living and Healthy Eating Among Older Canadians."

Osberg, Lars. "Economic Policy Variables and Population Health."

Polanyi, M., J. Eakin, J. Frank, H. Shannon and T. Sullivan. "Creating Healthier Work Environments: A Critical Review of the Health Impacts of Workplace Change."

Scott, K.A. "Balance as a Method to Promote Healthy Indigenous Communities."

Singer, Peter and Douglas K. Martin. "Improving Dying in Canada."

Steinhauer, Paul D. "Developing Resiliency in Children from Disadvantaged Populations."

Sudermann Marlies and Peter G. Jaffe. "Preventing Violence: School- and Community-Based Strategies."

Sullivan, T. , O. Uneke, J. Lavis, D. Hyatt and J. O'Grady. "Labour Adjustment Policy and Health: Considerations for a Changing World."

Tamblyn, Robyn and Robert Perreault. "Encouraging the Wise Use of Prescription Medication by Older Adults."

Wolfe, David A. "Prevention of Child Abuse and Neglect."

Zayed, Joseph and Luc Lefebvre. "Environmental Health: From Concept to Reality."

Striking a Balance Working Group

Arweiler, Delphine. "International Comparisons of Health Expenditures."

Brousselle, Astrid. "Controlling Health Care Costs: What Matters."

Deber, Raisa, Lutchmie Narine, Pat Baranek, Natasha Hilfer, Katya Masnyk Duvalko, Randi Zlotnik-Shaul, Peter Coyte, George Pink and A. Paul Williams. "The Public Private/Mix in Health Care."

Deber, Raisa and Bill Swan. "Puzzling Issues in Health Care Financing."

Fournier, Marc-André. "The Impact of Health Care Infrastructures and Human Resources on Health Expenditures."

Groupe de Recherche Interdisciplinaire en Santé. "How Canada's Health System Compares with that of Other Countries - An Overview."

Kennedy, Wendy. "Managing Pharmaceutical Expenditures: How Canada Compares."

Leibovich, Ellen, Howard Bergman and François Béland. "Health Care Expenditures and the Aging Population in Canada."

Marriott, John and Ann L. Mable. "Integrated Models: International Trends and Implications for Canada."

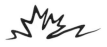

Maslove, Allan M. "National Goals and the Federal Role in Health Care."

Morgan, Steven G. "Issues for Canadian Pharmaceutical Policy."

Scott, Geoffroy. "International Comparison of the Hospital Sector."

Sullivan, Terrance. "Commentary on Health Care Expenditures, Social Spending and Health Status."

The Centre for International Statistics at the Canadian Council on Social Development. "Health Spending and Health Status: An International Comparison."

Evidence-Based Decision Making Working Group

Black, Charlyn. "Building a National Health Information Network."

Butcher, Robert. "Foundations for Evidence-Based Decision Making."

Fisher, Paul, Marcus J. Hollander, Thomas MacKenzie, Peter Kleinstiver, Irina Sladecek, and Gail Peterson. "Decision Support Tools in Health Care."

Kushner, Carol and Michael Rachlis. "Consumer Involvement in Health Policy Development." Tranmer, J.E., S. Squires, K. Brazil, J. Gerlach, J. Johnson, D. Muisner, B. Swan and Dr. R. Wilson. "Using Evidence-Based Decision Making: What Works, What Doesn't."